RISING

Fr

ASHES

Of

BENGAL'S
PARTITION

UNTOLD STORY OF A 'PHOENIX' ASPIRING
TO LIVE A NEW LIFE

JIBAN MUKHOPADHYAY

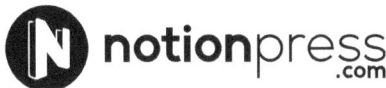

INDIA · SINGAPORE · MALAYSIA

Notion Press

Old No. 38, New No. 6
McNichols Road, Chetpet
Chennai - 600 031

First Published by Notion Press 2019
Copyright © Jiban Mukhopadhyay 2019
All Rights Reserved.

ISBN 978-1-64587-166-8

This book has been published with all efforts taken to make the material error-free after the consent of the author. However, the author and the publisher do not assume and hereby disclaim any liability to any party for any loss, damage, or disruption caused by errors or omissions, whether such errors or omissions result from negligence, accident, or any other cause.

While every effort has been made to avoid any mistake or omission, this publication is being sold on the condition and understanding that neither the author nor the publishers or printers would be liable in any manner to any person by reason of any mistake or omission in this publication or for any action taken or omitted to be taken or advice rendered or accepted on the basis of this work. For any defect in printing or binding the publishers will be liable only to replace the defective copy by another copy of this work then available.

Dedicated to my dear father, an enterprising man; the partition did not deter him, but ill health did; and to my mother, a soft and loving person, who would have lived longer, but for the partition. They would have been the happiest persons to read this humble story, if they were alive today.

Contents

Foreword

One of the privileges of my professional career has been the opportunity to meet and interact with a wide variety of other professionals. Apart from the osmosis of knowledge and perspectives due to such exposure, I also got to know a bit about the people I met. It has been a rewarding journey to know individuals. Within the first month of my joining Tata Sons Ltd in 1998, I received a note from DES (Department of Economics & Statistics) on the emerging WTO issues. WTO could impact Indian business and economy generally, and Tata companies specifically. Jiban Mukhopadhyay of DES, an Economics Think Tank of the Tata Group, had prepared the note. I found the note to be informative, insightful and focused on the business imperatives of the time.

At that time, I was chairing the Expert Committee on international Business and WTO of the Confederation of Indian Industry (CII). I had a discussion with Jiban and found him well versed both in academic as well as applied nuances of international business. I invited him to the next meeting of my committee in Delhi. Our relationship grew.

Having been born and grown up in Calcutta, I speak fluent Bengali. Jiban is an ethnic Bengali. Thus, we could vibe well on many things.

Under my overall supervision, Jiban and his team from DES worked out a strategic approach on global competitiveness related issues for the Tata Group companies. In this book, he briefly discusses this and several other issues, including what it meant to him to work in the Tata Group – its charismatic leaders and how the group practiced its unique business model of trusteeship. He was closely involved in working on a number of economic issues, inter alia, about the process of reform, restructuring, and the fast-emerging competitiveness of the Indian business and economy.

Jiban's book is something beyond the autobiographical, it provides a subaltern view of developments that he was witness to. He brings out a series of untold stories from his growing – up years in the post-partition Bengal to his navigating through torturous phases of life, spanning across seven decades. He reflects on his memory of events of his time, people and space. The story moves with socio-political, economic and historic canvas. He expands his horizon from Calcutta to Delhi and Mumbai.

It is a unique journey of a lone boy thrust into the ashes of Bengal's partition, battled on many fronts, who never got dejected. He moves, learns and puts down his experiences – always with a determined, albeit objective, optimism. This is the untold story of the striving and suffering of a generation.

I found it interesting that while discussing an event, he moves over to bringing certain relevant references from customs, practices, history, academics and all that. He draws illuminating inferences, puts down his considered personal views, in his book. For instance, when he makes an objective appraisal of the market-oriented reforms introduced in India since July 1991, he meticulously points out that in a large, poor country like India with so many complexities, there is need for an efficient and positive intervention of the Government in areas like health, education and certain physical infrastructure. He reads Milton Friedman and Friedrich Hayek carefully, but as a true Bengali his economic philosophy is left of center.

He moves over with spontaneity from long years of corporate culture to teaching in management school. He greatly enjoyed interacting with young minds of the future. He also makes a case about the need for developing a relevant curriculum for management education in India because of the country's unique reality.

R. Gopalakrishnan
Former director, Tata Sons Ltd, Mumbai

Preface

This is the story of the Partition's Generation – those who were born in Bengal a few years before or after India's Independence on August 15, 1947. Ironically, India was partitioned on this day.

The children of partition accepted the challenges arising out of the dreadful situation of being uprooted from their habitat and home in erstwhile East Pakistan, now Bangladesh. This is the story of their tears, their agonies as well as their determination and guts for taking up challenges of life.

This is not a sob story. This is the untold story of the unflinching determination of the Partition's Generation to move ahead. This is the story of their struggle for living, not just survival. This is the story of the real people – people who did not curse their fate and sit idle shedding tears. This is the story of the post-Partition Generation of Bengal, told by a protagonist of this generation.

The family of the narrator of this untold story – and many families of his close relatives, friends and million others – had to move over to partitioned India from East Pakistan. They all belonged to undivided India. Suddenly, they became aliens in their own home country and had to uproot themselves. They had been living and enjoying a reasonably comfortable lifestyle. Their demands were not too high. The alluvial soil was very fertile and food was available aplenty. There were festivals and ceremonies almost around the year. The overall societal condition was peaceful.

They did not know too many sophisticated occupational skills beyond the ones for running life and livelihood in the eastern part of Bengal. It was a sort of feudalistic society at a lower level equilibrium. Yet they were content with their simple life and living.

The people of Bengal were also not very enterprising. It was not required for them to be so. Nature had given them enough to lead their life.

The Governments, of India as well as West Bengal, also could not think of any innovative approach to give this vast mass of uprooted people an alternative approach to a new lifestyle. There was no proper plan for rehabilitating refugees. The supply of cash and food doles continued for many decades to millions who had to live in refugee camps.

Many refugees lived in camps. Many others occupied vacant lands, constructed buildings illegally and established colonies named after renowned leaders like Netaji Subhas, Gandhiji, Bagha Jatin and many others. They had to fight cops and goons hired by rich owners of those properties in a long drawn battle. Eventually, those who succeeded built their simple houses with ordinary and cheap materials like tin, straws, bamboos in and around Calcutta. That was a torturous journey.

The educated elderly persons with leadership quality organized themselves and started setting up schools for boys and girls. That was the starting point of building the future. It was from that base of education, the post-Partition Generation of boys and girls tried to move forward in life. Fortunately, the schools were subsequently aided by government fund.

Symbolically, this is a story of the Phoenixes. This is the story how they 'rose from the ashes with renewed youth to live through another cycle.'[1]

The story moves with time – over seven decades – around people and space in the socio-political, industrial and economic landscape of West Bengal as well as India.

The story unfolds uniqueness of many personalities, eminent as well as ordinary, lights and shades that the protagonist has come across in his checkered life. It moves from individuals to the community. It covers protagonist's student life in eminent educational institutions in West Bengal, exposure to the outer world of knowledge, his unenviable experience of working in the Planning Department of the Government of West Bengal and plight of the people in the economically weakest district of Bengal.

The story moves over to the protagonist's increasing exposure to the outside world, his joining the Tata Group's Economic Think Tank; it brings out personalities of some top business leaders and provides analysis of topical economic issues. It also focuses light and provides an insight into the process of economic reform, the paradigm shift in the economy and society in India, the globalization and the emerging competition, the restructuring of industries, the world of statistics, working with Government departments and lively story of a top management institute.

The author's experiences are as colorful as the kaleidoscopic movement of personalities and events in the societal space across time.

While navigating through the above, and more, the protagonist makes a humble attempt – like threading a garland – to track the checkered trajectory of the life's journey of the Freedom's, nay Partition's, Generation of Bengal.

This is an unknown and untold story. This is my story – our story, the story of our time, our space and our people.

I seek readers indulgence to say that I have been inspired by the unique style of James Joyce's Ulysses, '… the stream of consciousness'. Joyce wrote Ulysses depicting the thoughts and actions of its main characters, Leopold Bloom as well as Molly Bloom and others on a single ordinary day, June 16, 1904 in Dublin in a "…scattered and fragmented form similar to the way thoughts, perceptions and memories actually appear in our mind".[2]

I have tried to make my book a smooth read – well, as far as I could. I have made a humble effort to put down my thoughts in a sequential and somewhat orderly manner as they came in my mind when I was taking a 16-hour direct flight from JFK to Mumbai.

Jiban Mukhopadhyay,
Mumbai May 2019

Acknowledgments

This book has its genesis in a deep conversation between father and son some years ago in Pittsburgh. Somshuvra, my son, was doing his postdoctoral research in Carnegie Mellon University. I visited him. He was keen to know in detail about our – his – family, its heritage, history. He had already heard bits and pieces about it. He wanted to know the story in a chronological and comprehensive manner.

I gave him names and whatsoever details I knew of our last seven ancestors before my father. With that, I began the story. He interrupted me many times; asked pointed questions when I was not clear enough on some points. It was a long session well past midnight. Both of us had tears in our eyes when it was over.

He insisted that I must write down this story – the story of the Partition's Generation – of which I am a humble protagonist. That's how it all began. Unless he had asked and pursued me to do it, I might not have written it. Thank you Som.

In this journey, Tapati, my wife, is my travel partner – she also belongs to the post-Partition Generation. Lot of credit goes to her in shaping and reshaping the narration. Her father was a freedom fighter of repute, a 'Tamrapatra' recipient of the Government of India. Along with his friends, he established schools for boys and girls in several colonies in Jabalpur area of Calcutta. Tapati lived through those difficult real life experiences during her growing up years. I would not have been able to develop this story without her help.

I am grateful to Mr.R. Gopalakrishnan, former director, Tata Sons Ltd, and an eminent author himself for the encouragement and help in many ways. He also wrote the 'Forward' of my book, adding a huge value to my humble work.

Some of my close friends and colleagues helped and encouraged me. I had several rounds of discussion with Dr. Debasis Malik, professor (S.P. Jain Institute of Management and Research (SPJIMR), Mumbai about my experiences of my life. He encouraged me to write these experiences and provided support. I am thankful to him.

Bivash Chakraborty, a bright engineer having a critical, albeit critical mindset has not only read the text in a meticulous way but also given substantive suggestions. I also thank Shakti, my brother-in-law, for his support and encouragement.

My thanks go to Dr. Bhaskar Das, group president, Republic, Dr. Koustav Mazumdar, professor, SPJIMR and Arindam Duttgupta for their encouragement.

I thank Chinmoy Joshi, research associate, for rendering technical help on many occasions when I was stuck on my laptop. Thanks also go to Prajakta Jadav for technical help.

I take this opportunity to also thank the Management, Editors and other staff members of Notion Press for helping me publish this book.

I tried my best to take care of facts, informations and data. I have used real names of many persons with whom I have interacted and worked. I am grateful to them; they made my journey unto this life meaningful. In some cases, I have changed names due to obvious reasons.

Since the story belonged to the pre-Kolkata era, the city has been referred to as Calcutta in this narration.

Views and observations about people and facts are entirely my own.

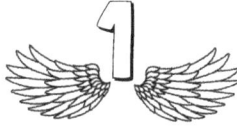

My Dream House is Gone!

I take my aisle seat in the front row of the economy class. There is no corporate account any longer. It is a 16-hour direct flight from JFK to Mumbai, a huge distance of 12,564 kms. It will be a backbreaking flight. Shutting my eyes, I take a deep breath and try to relax. Being half-dozy, I see images – kaleidoscopic images of my childhood home.

I just cannot erase the image of the mighty river Padma – with her extensive width, stretching up to the horizon, a cool sheet of light bluish water – gently rippling in the soft and gentle wind. There are large patches of sandbanks and tiny islands, called *chars* in Bengali, with occasional habitations. River Padma becomes very ferocious and destructive during the monsoon; it breaks one side of the bank, depending on the river's speed, volume of water it carries, its course and slope. The river has been changing its course and direction over the years.

It was sometime in early December in 2009 when I went to Dhaka, the capital of Bangladesh. My wife Tapati was doing an interdisciplinary research project as a SAARC Fellow under UGC Bangladesh and living in Dhaka for six months. I went there to be with her for two weeks.

She had already located and visited her father's ancestral home in Dhaka. The large three-storey building with two wings stands still even today. Two Muslim families occupy the house. Her father was a freedom fighter, spent over 12 years in British prison. She discussed with some prominent Bangladeshi friends about visiting my ancestral place in a village called Hasail in Tongibari (presently, a sub-district), Bikrampur (presently a pargana), Munshiganj district, Dhaka division. It would take four hours by road from Dhaka city.

I was very excited, at the same time scared. At last, I would be able to visit my ancestral home, my dream home, where I was born and lived for about four years before our family moved to Calcutta (now Kolkata) a few months before India's Independence – and the partition of India.

What memory could a four-year-old child have? Perhaps some patches of images here and there. Some sights and sounds. Some tunes. Some happy feelings. Some smiles and joys. Some agonies. Some scary thoughts. Some frights.

However, the stories I heard so often about the house, the place, the village and the habitat from my relatives, who would not stop talking about their ancestral home. They had to uproot themselves suddenly from their home of generations. Gruesome communal riots went on for several days affecting many parts of Bengal and Punjab, killing thousands, and thousands.

One early morning a large number of people found themselves as aliens in their own country!

I heard many stories, anecdotes from many of my close relatives. I witnessed continuous flow of tears from my mother, grandmother, aunts and many relatives, who could never forget their easy-going lifestyle in their villages, which they had to leave behind. As a child, I could not understand why we had to leave our home. I could not understand why we have to live in such poor conditions after coming to Calcutta. Why sometimes we had to miss one, or the other meal of the day?

However, in my own small way I realized that time was bad. Besides, my father was suffering from something like a Parkinson's disease since his early 30s. An enterprising person was not in his best physical form at the time of partition.

The image of the home that we left used to haunt me day and night. I made the picture of my 'home' mixed with collages of stories I heard from so many people, colored with my imagination and my own memory, from the dream that I so often used to have. When I told about my dream home to my mother, she confirmed the description of my dream home.

Bikrampur is a low-lying area. People have to walk miles on narrow, circuitous and untarred roads across fields. In the monsoon, the area would be largely under water. Houses in certain low-lying areas have been built on raised wooden platforms. People had to move on small country boats during rainy season. Because of this problem, farming was limited. People took up education in cities and were employed there for their livelihood. Those who used to work in big cities like Dhaka or Calcutta used to visit their villages during holidays like Durga Puja. Those who used to work close by smaller towns used to visit home during weekends. Bikrampur was sort of a money order economy.

Bikrampur, being a place for relatively well off and educated people, contributed many important and historically famous Bengalis. There used to be many distinguished villages in Bikrampur. Ours was one of them. It had a prominent place in the history of Bengal, now Bangladesh. Our house in Hasail was located near a canal, close to the eastern bank of the mighty river Padma.

I remember from the patches of my childhood memory – seeing my father getting down from the boat. He was a tall, fair complexioned and handsome person. He brought many household goods and gifts for us. He worked somewhere and used to come home occasionally. A crowd of relatives and friends stood there to welcome him. I could see my mother looking out from the window.

The road leading to the gate of the house had rows of various trees on both the sides, creating a kind of a canopy. There were trees of *hortoki, amlaki, bel, jamrul, kalojam, golupjam, chelta, aata, falsa,* and, of course, mangoes, jackfruit and guava. We had several varieties of mango trees. There was a very tall mango tree on the left side of our house. I heard that the mango from this tree was very large and looked magnificent. However, it smelled foul and tasted bad!

On the right side, there was a large pond, covered on all four sides by short and bushy trees. Even in the mid-day, the pond's water looked dark black. There were some bushy and short sized mango plants, growing very tiny and red colored mangos. These mangos had even tinnier seeds and tasted delicious. I have never seen such varieties of mango anywhere. There was also another mango tree just behind our main house. It used to bear only a few gorgeous red colored mangoes in the season, delicious and very sweet, so much, so it was *Bou Pagla* – if a new bride tastes it, she would go mad with joy! No one could tell me why it was named so absurdly. There were a few *karamcha* (cherry fruits of Bengal) bushes with small fruits of riotously red and white color, covered by their thick and glossy green leaves. It looked magnificent.

Our house faced a narrow road. The road from the canal ended almost at the entrance of our house. There was a railing alongside two central pillars on the front verandah. The kitchen was separate, behind the main house. There was no electricity. Kids were served their supper when the small flowers of *sandhyamoni* (evening star) and the tiny and yellow *jhinge* (ridge gourd) flowers blossomed in the twilight – soon it would be dark. Pitch dark. There were no electric power – only kerosene lanterns or lamps.

Behind the kitchen was a smaller pond, with a path between the two ponds. The narrow path would lead you to the orchard, maintained not in very sophisticated style; it looked natural. There were some vegetable patches here and there.

My grandmother was the overall supervisor. She had a number of helping hands. I heard that she loved and took care of the plants like her own kids; she used to fondle them, talk to them, and see that they grow in a balanced way so that their flowers and fruits could grow in good shape.

My grandfather was very fond of growing fruits and flowers. He created the orchard. Typical flowers of Bengal like *otoshi, karobi, tagar, sandhamoni, dopati, jaba* of heavenly colors, *shephali and gandharaj* were scattered around the house. There were also some creepers with various shades of *aparajita* and *madhabilata*. Nature took good care of the beauty of the landscape.

Our house and the plot of land were on the southeastern corner leading from the road. On our left side, there were houses of two close relatives. In between was a huge open space, a courtyard. Layered periodically with cow dung, it would not be muddy even after heavy rain. It was neat, clean and shiny. During harvesting time, crops used to be cleaned, processed and preserved on the courtyard.

Standing on the bank of the mighty river Padma, I was speechless. Tapati was nearby. She too was silent, allowing me to absorb the visual impact of the great river. Sure, she knew exactly what was happening in my mind.

Some people were standing there. I wanted to see my dream home. The people around were speechless. Nobody spoke a word. We went to the nearby Hasail *Bazaar,* where the message of our arrival had already reached. A couple of shop owners, Tapan babu and Nandi babu invited us to sit and offered cold drinks and fruits. They knew about our *Mukherjee Bari.* Nandi was born in 1946, about time when our family left the village for Calcutta as partition was imminent. He told us that he had heard from his elders about our family. He told us that there was a library, probably run by our family. Bipin Pal, headmaster of Banari Para High School, was out of station. He called the next day and invited us for another visit and lunch. He also had heard about our family and house. They all appreciated my wife's initiative to come and visit her father-in-law's house. After all, the village's *bahu* (daughter-in-law) had come! What a warm welcome to both us!

I was getting restless. Over six decades had passed. Things must have changed beyond recognition. Have I done right to visit my dream home?

I asked the people around impatiently where my home was. There was a hesitation. Nobody opened up for quite some time. I guessed there was something wrong. I also became silent and looked at the faces around me, one by one. Every one avoided eye contact. My mind shouted inside. Where is my dream house? Silence continued. Tapati held my hand tightly.

Eventually, Tapan babu came close to me, took my hands into his and told me that the ferocious river Padma had engulfed our house and several other houses some years ago. It had been mercilessly breaking and submerging the land and properties on the eastern bank. It had been changing its course sidewise. In winter, it looked cool, calm, and beautiful like the smiling Durga Mata as it is now. However, the monsoon transforms the Padma into a fearsome and destructive mother Kali. Tapan babu pointed out the area in the Padma where once my dream house stood. I looked at the area; for me it was no different from the vast, softly rippling miles of water! My dream house lay underneath!

I could not believe my ears. A blend of agony, anger, frustration and sadness overwhelmed my mind. I stood there for several minutes like a piece of stone. Tapati held my hands tight. Tears flowed from our eyes. I could not utter any word for quite some time.

I heard from my father that his ancestors moved to this place in Hasail from some other place where their house and properties were also submerged by the river Padma. However, that was several generations ago. This was the second time in a few generations again our properties were submerged. How many times should we become homeless?

I could not register in my brain anything that some elderly people said to console me. I stood there like a statue. My mind travelled far away to the images that I had cultivated for so long.

Soon I realized I had to take the initiative to rationalize my mind and take charge of the situation.

I thanked them for their nice words, which came from their heart. They had tears in their eyes. Many held my hands and said comforting words. I was happy to know these poor people with golden hearts. Tapati spoke to them more intimately. She has this trait. After a few moments, I felt relieved. What I would have seen most probably could be a dilapidated structure, poorly maintained and occupied by others, which would be far away from my dream house. At least my dream house remained in my mind.

Standing transfixed on the unbelievably cool and vast Padma, it was difficult for me to accept that this great peaceful looking river of today would be so ferocious and with such destructive power during the monsoon! I heard stories from the people standing around us that such incidents happened so often during the monsoon. Poor people construct light and movable houses here. When they hear the sound of the river gorging with huge ferocity, neighbors come together to physically move their houses to a relatively safe and distant place. Later on, they would occupy the land on the *chars*.

They asked us, seriously, in case we are interested, they would help us to get some land on the *chars*. So nice of them! Obviously, we were not interested.

My mind moved over to what I heard from my father and some other close relatives. There are many incidents, which are difficult to be explained by a rational mind, with a scientific temperament. Yet I must mention what I heard.

I recall that one night there was a shrill cry and noise from one of our neighbor's house at some distance, which was attacked by rioters. People had been crying and asking for help. There were sounds of gunshots. Several people known to my family were killed, their house looted. We were hiding under the bed. Perhaps, some young girls were raped before they were killed. In the jungle wild animals kill for food or when attacked. They never rape and then kill. Human beings are sometimes worse than animals. This is not the rule or order of nature. Guess, in normal times people are good-natured like Dr. Jekyll. But, the same people get transformed to Mr. Hyde when the time is abnormal, charged with unrest and hatred.

I am not going to provide any socio-psychological explanation about why riots do take place, or why the aggrieved section of one community wants to attack the other, or vice versa, due to some historic misdoings by their distant ancestors in the past. The shrieking cry for help, the sound of the gunshots, and the loud laughter of the rioters still haunt my ears. As a kid, I did not understand why such atrocity had to happen. Why people belonging to one religion would kill people belonging to another?

A few days later a Muslim friend from the neighborhood came to my father and told that we would be safe and there would not be any attack on us. However, my father and other relatives decided to move over to Calcutta soon. Independence of India meant homelessness, rape and murder for millions in Bengal and Punjab. Both the communities were affected adversely, some more, some less.

I have heard that my father had sold or leased the main residential part of the house to his close Muslim friend for a modest amount. He offered to take care of the house and other properties in our absence. He would return the house, if we ever decided to return. Sure, a very friendly deal as it looked; if we do not return, then he got not only the house but also all our properties for a pittance. In any disaster, there are some losers and some gainers.

But this is not the story, this is just the background of the story of a supernatural, if I may say so, event.

On the day the Muslim gentleman came to take the possession of the house, he could not enter. Two large snakes came from nowhere and they circled around the two pillars, one snake each on one pillar. The snakes made hissing noises, swinging their hoods vigorously and were on attacking postures. I was told that these two snakes, husband and wife, are our house guards. As the local legend goes, these snakes are known as *bastusaps,* who guard the house.

Then my grandmother, aunt and my mother came forward with two bowls of milk and placed them in front of the two large snakes. They cooled down by seeing my grandmother, aunt and my mother approaching. The snakes knew them well. In rural Bengal, particularly in the east, snakes are associated with the mythological deity, *Manasa.* Snakes are not harmed under normal circumstances.

Looking back today, I am amazed to see how people in those days in rural Bengal, particularly in the east, lived in peace and harmony with nature. The land was very fertile and food used to grow aplenty almost on its own. People had warm relations with the folks around; cattle were reared with love and care. Cats, dogs, birds, even snakes and insects were part of the living eco-system. It was a peaceful equilibrium embedded in the true spirit of Nature. We may call it primitive lifestyle in our so-called civilized societal living standard of today, with so many sophisticated and ever-changing high-tech gadgets, high-speed movement and luxurious living for those who can afford. These folks of my ancestors' generation in rural East Bengal were contented people without greed. They possessed certain fundamental human qualities and values. They co-existed harmoniously along with their surroundings, rich flora, fauna and the friendly animal world.

They sat in front of the snakes as if they were sitting before some deities, said some prayer with folded hands and addressed the snakes explaining under what compelling circumstances we would be leaving this house. With flowing tears in their eyes, they profusely thanked the snakes for guarding our house for generations and requested them to allow the new owner to enter.

Surprisingly, the snakes slowly came down from the pillars, slightly dipped their hoods in the milk container but did not sip, looked around with sad eyes at my grandmother and others by turning the hoods, and very slowly moved out, often looking back. Soon they were gone.

Another shock and surprise! When the snakes eventually disappeared, suddenly the flock of pigeons, living on the outer side of the building for generations, and was very much a part of the family, flew away. Flapping of their wings made a loud and eerie sound. It happened so suddenly! Everyone in the gathering stood still with folded hands and saying prayers in local tongue. Their eyes were filled with flowing tears. A bad omen! Pigeons were friends of happy times. They would not stay if times were not good.

I knew my family's bad time had come.

CHAPTER 2

Going Back to the Roots

The route map on the screen shows a semi-circular path. Since the earth is spherical, the shortest distance between two points on a sphere is an arc, and not a straight line; the arc is the 'Great Circle Route.'

My core family was composed of my grandmother, an aunt – my father's widowed elder sister, my mother and father. My father was working in Barisal district. I did not see my grandfather – Mahesh Chandra. I was born long after he died. He was managing an estate in the south – eastern part of Bengal owned by a *Raja* (rich and powerful *zamindar*) based in Calcutta. My grandmother, Suvashini, was tall and slim, a very formidable lady, with a strong personality. She had the courage to defy the societal custom even in those orthodox days.

In those years, *Brahmins* belonging to *Radi Shreni* – the *Kuleen Brahmins* – supposedly were at the top of the pyramid of the caste system. Four categories of *Kuleen* Brahmins are with surnames, Mukhopadhyay, Bandopadhyay, Chattopadhyay and Gangopadhyay. The then Bengal King – Ballal Sen of Sen Dynasty supposedly gave this recognition.[1] King Lakshman Sen modified this system sometime during the 12th century. Incidentally, Mukherjee, Banerjee, Chatterjee and Ganguly are the Anglicized version of the four surnames mentioned above. English tongues could not pronounce the original surnames.

There is another category of Brahmins, called *Vaidik Brahmins*, usually with surnames like Bhattacharyays and Chakrabortys. They are supposed to be well versed in Vedic literature and rituals. They claim to be in the top category of Brahmins. They performed rituals even in the houses of the *Radi Shreni Brahmins*. There are also certain other categories of Brahmins like *Barendra Brahmins* with surnames like Sanyal and Bagchi.

Alongside, there was *Kuleen Kayasthyas*, with surnames like Ghosh, Bose, Guha and Mitra. They were the prosperous class being involved in business and trading. Besides, there was Vaidyas like Senguptas and Dasguptas, specializing in medicine and medical treatment.

These were the top categories in the complex caste system, introduced over a thousand years ago, in Bengal.

According to one view, King Adisura of Sura dynasty originally brought the Kuleen Brahmins to Bengal in the mid-10th century from Kannyakubja, Kannauj in today's central India, to enhance brahminical culture. It is a long, complex and convoluted history of Bengali caste and social system, whose authenticity is difficult to establish. In this context, it is important to note that the kingdom of the Sen Dynasty was said to be in *Bikrampur*, christened then as *Shribikrampur*. [2]

Radi Shreni Brahmins are divided into 36 *Mels* (groups). Marriage had to happen within the small group of a particular *Mel* of *Kuleen* Brahmins, and not outside. As a result, many such Brahmin males had to indulge in large number of marriages. One reason of such odd practice could be demographic imbalance, with more girls and less males among the *Kuleen* Brahmins of a particular *Mel*. As such, even very old men with fragile health belonging to this group of *Kuleen* Brahmins used to marry large numbers of young girls.

Noted Bengali author Kamal Kumar Mazumdar (1914–1979) wrote in his striking novel, *Antarjwali Jatra* (The Final Passage, 1962) [3] about this atrocious practice of '*ghat* murder'. Mazumdar's story is about an erudite old man Sitaram, who was taken to the bank of the river Ganga so that he would fast unto his death. However, to the discomfort of his relatives he survived for long. An astrologer predicted that Sitaram would not die alone. He persuaded Sitaram to get married. When he would die, his wife would join him to the funeral pyre and be a *Sati*. Thus, both would reach heaven!

The mischievous astrologer arranged to get a greedy and heartless Brahmin, who came with his beautiful young and unmarried daughter, Yashovati. The Brahmin forced his daughter to get married to Sitaram.

The orthodox thinking was that a *Sati* would bring honor to the family. Indeed, Sitaram got married to Yashovati. Goutam Ghose made a touching, albeit morbid, national award winning movie on this story in 1987.

Orthodox belief was that if the *Kuleen* Brahmin daughters were not married early, the family would incur a 'sin', and would go to hell after death! After marriage, a girl would mostly stay in her father's family, creating many tensions, while the husbands, who married *N* – number of girls, taking dowry, would move from one in-law's family to another, visiting perhaps as a guest, and thus supporting his livelihood. It was an evil and obnoxious system.

My grandmother defied this evil system and married off her two daughters to non-*Kuleen Brahmins*. Such action used to invite punishment from the so-called society (*Samaj*), e.g., *Kuleens were* downgraded *to Bhanga* (broken) *Kuleen* status.

My aunt, Suniti, was my father's second eldest sister. She became a widow at an early age of about 15. She was a very beautiful person. Her young husband was studying medicine. The bright young man died early due to cholera, for which there was no treatment then. As was the practice, my grandfather brought Suniti back home. She would have to lead a highly disciplined life as a Brahmin widow, eating strictly vegetarian food of certain types, this too only once a day. The restriction was to ensure she lived a sort of pious life! There was no question of remarriage, even though law permitted it then.

Pandit Ishwar Chandra Vidyasagar (1820–1891), a giant among social reformers, educationist and a litterateur, was desperate to stop the evil system of polygamy practiced by the *Kuleen Brahmins*. He took a leading role in facilitating the enactment of the Widow Remarriage Act, enacted by the British East India Company on July 25, 1856. Despite this enactment, not too many widow remarriages took place. Even in the mid-20th century, the widow remarriage was a taboo!

Another evil, brutal and criminal practice was *Sati Daaha*. A married young Brahmin woman, whose husband died, was forced to dress like a bride and then was forced by the so-called relatives and friends to join the dead husband on the flaming pyre. I have mentioned the disgusting story of Sitaram above.

Raja Ram Mohan Roy (1772–1833), a highly erudite person, a great social and religious reformer, persuaded, inter alia, the British East India Company to enact a law to stop this brutal system of *Sati Daaha* as early as 1829, over a quarter century before enacting the Widow Remarriage Act. It was enforced in the territories ruled by company. Queen Victoria uniformly enacted it for the whole of British India in 1861. Thereafter, it took 127 years for the Indian Parliament to enact The Commission of Sati (Prevention) Act, 1897 in 1988!

Orthodoxy still prevails in certain sections among our people. Why, in the Western Express Highway near Malad East, Mumbai, there is flyover named 'Rani Sati Flyover'! There also is Rani Sati Marg adjacent to the flyover. The regional passport office of Government of India is located on this road.

As was the practice, my grandfather delegated the responsibility of managing the family affairs to my widowed aunt. Perhaps, the practice was introduced for the mental engagement of the deprived young widow. Thus, my aunt was the high command in the family. Though she took care of everybody and was affectionate to all, she was a dominating personality. She made my mother's life extremely difficult by bossing over her.

My mother, Usha, was a very soft spoken and nice person. Her complexion was very smooth, not very fair, and not too dark at all. Her height was medium. She had locks of black hair. She had large eyes with a serene smile. Everybody used to like her. But she was not allowed to take charge of her family, thanks to my aunt's tight grip over everything. I knew my mother did not like the high command, but she did not make it an issue.

My father, Santosh Kumar, was a tall, fair complexioned and handsome person. I did not understand under what circumstances a very rich but childless *Zamindar* family adopted him. While he was doing his matriculation examination, young Santosh had to return home at the instance of my dominating aunt. Because of the family pressure after the death of my grandfather, he had to take up a job and could not complete his education. He did not openly reveal his mental grief at not being able to complete his education. However, he learned to read and write reasonably good English. He was well versed in real estate business practices and law.

My father was also working in a *Raj* estate in Barisal district as a 'treasurer', working for the rich *zamindars* based in Calcutta. Our family was well off. Several families of our close relatives depended on my father's financial help.

My father's eldest sister, Hemabala, was married to Upendra Chakraborty, a forest officer, working in Assam. He was smart with guns; he could shoot down a flying bird. They used to live in a nearby village, *Routbhog*, with large landed property. They were very well off.

My father's third elder sister, Labannyabala, was married to Sudhannay Ranjan Mallick, living in Purasar, Tangibari. She died soon after her marriage. But her husband's wife by second marriage almost replaced my biological aunt, both by her beautiful look and sweet behavior. The youngest sister of my father, Subarna, was married to Makhanlal Khasnobis, who was a teacher, living in *Paikpara*.

All of them were living within a short radial distance in various villages from our village Hasial. Besides, there were many relatives living in adjacent villages. It was happy and vibrant community living in close togetherness sharing their smiles and joys as well as tears and sorrows. The partition of India broke this age-old harmony of living together.

My mother, Usha, came from a small village called *Dhoprapasa*, under the postal jurisdiction of *Swarnagram*, and a well-known village. My maternal grandfather, Jagadish Chandra Bhattacharyay, also died before I was born. Professionally, he used to be the manager of legal and related issues of the local *zamindar*. The family was well off. Every year Durga Puja and Kali Puja were organized by the family.

My *mama* (maternal uncle), Ratan, was five years older to me. He had a clear memory about our leaving home. He helped me with details of life in the then eastern part of Bengal

I have three maternal aunts. The eldest, Lakshmi, became a widow at an early age like my Suniti aunt. She used to stay with her husband's family, occasionally visiting her mother's house. My maternal grandmother, Surabala, was a very religious and orthodox person. If she touched fish even by accident, she had to take a full bath. My second aunt, Asha, was married to a cop, a nice but short-tempered person. The youngest aunt, Sati, was married to Jiban Bandhu Chakraborty, my namesake, was initially working in military service, later with a shipping company after moving to Calcutta.

With quite a number of aunts from both sides, uncles as well, I am privileged to have a battalion of cousins. Counting my father's cousins and their children, the number was very large. I was lucky to have enjoyed the love and affection of my elder cousins.

My *mamabari* in *Dhorapasha* was close to a medium sized pond, with its surface water almost touching the ground level. At times, this created lots of fun as well as accidents. Sometimes during rains, certain types of fishes like *kai* used to 'walk' up on the ground. They used their fangs to jump forward. It was fun among children, who could catch many fishes. Older boys and girls had a greater advantage. My skill was on the low side on such things. When it rained heavily and for long, the pond water used to rise and come close to the house bringing several varieties of small and tasty sweet water fishes. Our elders would catch those fishes with a hand made net.

Fishes in the pond, vegetables in the kitchen garden, fruits in trees, food grains in the adjacent fields – it was like an evolved version of food gatherers economy. Both the Hindu and Muslim communities without any hassle drew water from the pond. The two communities lived in harmony.

Sometimes, kids used to fall in the pond. They were always rescued. Almost everybody could swim. It used to be a contented living. Nature was very benevolent to people, making them easygoing. As such, the spirit of entrepreneurship did not develop.

The houses of my maternal relatives were spacious, though made of thick mud walls with straws or tins on the four-sided roofs. It was reasonably cool and comfortable inside. There were small hole like windows. I used to look through these holes and see the far away trees lining a huge playground. It was like watching a silent movie, when a football or a kabaddi game was going on. It was like seeing a movie from a long distance balcony; as if some otherworldly game was being played. Rather than going there and play, I used to enjoy the moving picture of the game. These environmentally compatible comfortable houses evolved over a long period.

Once there was a mild earthquake. I remember that water started moving up towards the house and going back and forth for several minutes. The trees were moving madly in the air. Ladies blew the *shankha* (conch shell) to warn people about the earthquake. It was, I think, a kind of an old-fashioned communication system informing and cautioning neighbors about an earthquake or such other calamities. It was also for praying to God.

There was a school in *Swarnagram* across the playground. My grand uncle was a teacher in this school. My *mama* used to study there. I heard stories of the formidable headmaster. He would go around the school with a cane in hand. He used the cane as a symbol of dispensing discipline and not as an instrument of delivering punishment. He quietly inspired senior students to join the freedom movement. The history of armed freedom struggle originating from Bengal has glowingly written about many such dedicated teachers.

While on this, I do not want to say that everything was great in the past. It was not. However, life was not stiffly competitive those years. It was a kind of lower level equilibrium. The problems in those days were at a different level, with lesser intensity. People used to live a contented life, with not too many demands, not too many gadgets. It was not a consumerist society. Perhaps, it was more sustainable model of living compared to today's complex, highly competitive and consumption=oriented lifestyle. All this was completely devastated after partition.

My close and extended families – and many, many more – migrated to West Bengal immediately after the partition largely because of the fear that Hindus were not safe in the place of their birth where they had been living from generations. This was the curse of the partition of India to millions of people. My family was not alone.

There were riots on both sides of Bengal. Muslims in the eastern side were killing Hindus, raping their girls, ransacking and occupying their houses and properties. In the west, too Hindus were killing Muslims. There was a complete breakdown of law and order for some time before, at the time of, as well as immediately after the partition.

Several millions of Hindus moved over a period, particularly immediately after the partition, to Calcutta and its adjacent areas, leaving their home for generations. Muslims also moved, albeit in much lesser numbers, from the western side to the east, which became their own State. What a massive uprooting!

CHAPTER

3

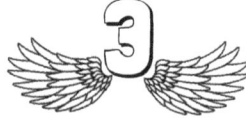

Something Incredibly Sad Has Happened

The flight map on the video screen is in front of me – we are about to fly over the vast North Atlantic Ocean. Pitch dark night outside. The map shows day light in certain other parts of the globe. Concept of time is so relative! I shut my eyes and try to put a thread to my thoughts.

I remember we were in a steamer, slowly moving towards a small port-town, Goalanda Ghat. I enjoyed the ride by the steamer, standing near the railing and looking at the flow of water churned out by the small propeller. I heard from seniors that we would take a train from Goalanda Ghat to Calcutta.

I do not have a full connect. However, I remember that after a long journey by train, we came to a small town called Ranaghat, 73 kms from Calcutta. It was evening. We had our dinner, my first eating out in a 'restaurant', rice and prawn curry. I enjoyed the meal. I did not know at that time what was in store for us.

I overheard my folks talking. People in thousands were leaving their home and habitat for generations, vaguely thinking that it was for a short period. Things would be sorted out by leaders like Gandhiji, Nehru, Jinnah, Patel and et al. For how long would they have to stay in India? Would they be able to return? Where would they stay in India? What would they do for a living? Where was Netaji Subhas? Was he not aware of what was happening to them? Why was he not there? Sure, he would come soon and resolve the issue.

Looking back, I think it was good that they had some hope of coming back to their age-old habitat. If that hope were not there, most of them would have been thoroughly devastated.

I asked my *mama* why we were going and where. He could not answer me clearly. He just said that our lives were in danger in East Bengal. We might return after sometime. Actually, he was happy that we were going to Calcutta. Going to Calcutta to study and live was a dream for young people. Calcutta is gorgeous. Bengali renaissance took place from Calcutta. It is the seat of education, art culture and literature. The soul of Bengal is charged with political activities. It is the city of protest, the city of activism. Above all, there is electricity, running water and in-house toilet. It is '*Kollolini Kolkata*' *(sound of* roaring waves)! Living in villages is no good. *Mama* told me that he heard that from one of his teachers, who came back from Calcutta recently to teach in the school. He did not like living in a village. *Mama* has started dreaming about going to Calcutta. I liked his confidence and happy voice.

My father and my aunt Sunitibala had already gone to Calcutta for my father's treatment. During the last one year, my father was not well. He was home and not going to work in Barisal. He was taking medicines. He was also practicing handwriting. His hand used to shake. So did his legs when walking. My mother was nursing him. I asked her what was wrong with my father. Mother held me close to her and said that he would be all right soon. I was delighted. However, there was always a doubt in my mind. When I closely looked at his face, he appeared sad and morose. Would he be cured and get back to his energetic self?

I remember the year my father took my mother, my sister Uma and me with him to his work place in Bahadurpur, Barisal. I remember we had a great time in the new place; my life's first, and the last, going out for a vacation with my core family. That was our first and last vacation together. That I did not know then.

Sitting quietly in one corner of the steamer and looking at the vast sheet of water of the river and amidst the sound of the rolling propeller my mind went back to my first ever family vacation of my little life. It was also the last.

I remembered the journey to Bahadurpur by boat like seeing age-old shots of a movie. In some parts of the river where the water level was low, the boat had to be dragged by rope. Two boatmen had to tie the boat with a long and sturdy rope and they would walk dragging the boat. It happened several times. Once I also got down with them. The boatmen moved too fast for my little paces. One of them happily carried me on his shoulder. I had a great joy ride.

It was immediately after monsoon and roads were submerged under water. People used to move by a tiny boat called *dingi* made of trunks of palm trees. One has to sit carefully and maintain balance; otherwise, it would turn upside down. It is a bicycle on water. If you would like to live in East Bengal, it was necessary to know swimming. One young person, working under my father, Haran da, took me out and helped me with the *dingi*.

Soon I was able to manage a trip by a d*ingi* on my own. Haran da remained always alert and watchful. It was great fun to move fast on a *dingi*, rowing with a flat and light piece of wood. I never had such a pleasure trip.

Haran da told me so many stories about life in that part of Bengal – about snakes biting people and thieves digging short tunnels inside the house to steal things at night. They would put huge quantity of oil on their bare bodies so that they could slip away if caught. They would eat, if some food was there, perhaps defecate, and then slip away with the stolen things through the narrow tunnel they had just made.

My father was not well. He was just recovering from typhoid. My mother used to make chicken soup every day in the afternoon for my father in a kerosene stove. I can still hear the hissing noise and see the blue flame of the stove. The doctor advised my father to take chicken soup. For us *Brahmins* eating chicken was a taboo. It would have been impossible to cook and consume chicken soup in Hasail. We would have been outcaste. In a less populated remote place in this part of the world, having chicken was safe. Haran da told me not to discuss this when we would go back to Hasail.

I remember two incidents taking place in Barisal in which I was involved. Once near a huge pond my sister Uma, slipped from the steps in the water. She was about to be drowned. I saw froth started coming out of her mouth. She was not too far from the cemented steps leading to water.

I was young, but thanks to Haran da's training, I could manage to swim, but I was not an expert. He told me that swimming is like walking on water. We walk on the land and swim in the water. In certain low-lying parts of East Bengal like Barisal or Bikrampur the saying was that people move by *Pao* and *Nao*, meaning that during dry season people walk on the road and during monsoon when most of the land mass is water logged, they move by boats. There was no other mode of transport.

I immediately got into the water and somehow dragged her near the steps. She was not too far off. By then Haran da was there and my sister was lifted on the shore. If Haran da did not arrive on time, both of us would have been under water forever.

The second incident was funny. I feel embarrassed even remembering it. One early morning just before the sunrise, I started nagging that I must have *kai* fish curry and rice. It was impossible to persuade me. My mother told me that she would serve it with lunch. I started howling. Haran da was already awake. He came, watched the drama, and told my mother not to worry. I came to know later that live *kai, magur* and *shing* fishes were preserved in a large earthen pot with water for emergency purpose. He got some *kai* fish, lit the stove and helped my mother to make the curry and rice. By then I went back to sleep. Whenever there was any discussion about my stubbornness, I had to hear this story many times.

The memory of our sweet *Barisal* trip is still on my mind.

We came to Chandannagar, the town that was under French domination. We were together with my maternal uncle's folks – a lot of them. My Lakshmi aunt had some connection with Chandannagar. Lakshmi aunt became a widow at an early age; it was good that her late husband's family took care of her. She did not have to come back to her father's family after being a widow as my paternal aunt had to. The family had some properties in Chandannagar. This was the reason for us to land in Chandannagar.

We stayed there for a couple of weeks. My father arrived after a few days; and our family – my grandmother, aunt, mother, sister and me – moved to Calcutta.

We moved to 18, Mahim Halder Street, Kalighat. It was a vacant plot, next to a three-storey red building, which stands there even today. The plot was behind the house of the landlord, next to where Durga Puja of Forward Club used to take place on Hazra road side. Close to it, there was the Kalighat Fire Brigade building. On Sunday mornings, the fire brigade people used to do mock firefighting drills. It used to be quite a spectacle to watch their exercise. The fire brigade building stands there even today. There used to be a narrow brick-made lane from the fire brigade building on Hazra Road side connecting Mahim Haldar Street. Immediately opposite our makeshift dwelling on Mahim Haldar Street, there was an empty ground, a congested slum thereafter. A narrow road ran through the slum reaching Kali Temple Road. The famous Ma Kali's temple was less than 10 minutes' walk from our place.

Today Harish Mukherjee Road has passed through these three plots, and stretches straight up to the Kali temple.

My father made a make-shift dwelling on this plot where we all moved. In the front, adjacent to the road was my father's tiny business 'enterprise', fuel wood agency, selling fuel wood and some stationery goods. There was a coconut tree in the right front corner, where a small rectangular signboard with the name of the shop used to hang. Over a short period, his tiny business generated sufficient resources for us to live. My father, despite his ill health, was an enterprising and independent-minded person.

We had a reasonably good time for a couple of years. I got admission in Kalighat Mahakali Patshala in the junior KG level. Today it is a junior college for girls. This was my first formal schooling. Prior to this, I had a home tutor. Subsequently, I got admission to first standard in Kalighat High School. Both schools were close to our place, a short walking distance.

I have some small memories about the second school. I remember our drill sir, who was a tough but an affectionate teacher. He used to shout a lot, but never hit or harassed any student. I developed a close friendship with one classmate, Biren, living near Patua Para, on the other side of Hazra Road, where idols are made even today. Our friendship developed under a peculiar circumstance. An argument between Biren and I led to an exchange of blows and wrestling on the school ground. The drill sir was there. He rushed in and separated us. He wiped our dirt from our uniforms and body. He smiled and said, "Sometime fighting is good". Now you two boys shake hands thrice and say loudly, "We are friends." We did so. "Do not ever fight," he said. "Hold your hands and go. I'm watching." We did the same and smiled at each other. The drill sir came forward, smiled and patted our backs. We became friends since then. I lost contact with him when we moved out from Calcutta.

I often remember the incident. During my later years, I also taught in a school. When I was a teacher, I fondly remembered our drill sir. He became my model in handling students, with love and care, yet being tough, depending on the situation.

I remember two incidents that happened during our stay in Kalighat. One was relating to India's Independence Day, August 15, 1947. My Bhanbaranjan uncle rented an open truck. About eight/10 persons, including me, enjoyed a ride across the streets of Calcutta throughout the day. Every street entrance was decorated with flowers. There were colorful *pandols*. People sang patriotic songs and danced around. There was celebration all around. India at last is an Independent country – well two separate countries, India and Pakistan.

In the evening, we went near Beliaghata where Mahatma Gandhi had been staying in Hyderi Manzil. He came to the city in the wake of the large-scale riot-ridden violence, which preceded the independence/partition.

Gandhiji did fast on the day of Independence. He did not celebrate as he thought that '… the kind of freedom we have got today contains also the seeds of future conflict between India and Pakistan'. He was right.

After Gandhiji's arrival in Calcutta a week before the Independence Day, he tried to persuade both the communities to live in peace. He was not successful initially. He started an indefinite fast from September 1. Eventually, on September 4, representatives of both Hindu and Muslim communities surrendered weapons and pledged before him to stop violence.

The city suffered a riot beginning on August 16, 1946, the 'Direct Action Day' announced by the Muslim League Council. A massive manslaughter followed between Hindu and Muslim communities.

Gandhiji also went to Noakhali, in East Bengal, where a massive rioting was going on during October and November 1946. Gandhiji stayed in Noakhali for bringing peace to the riot-affected areas. An estimated number of 5,000 to 10,000 people (exact number not known) from Hindu community were killed in the riot. Gandhiji used to walk through roads of towns and villages to spread messages of peace and non-violence. However, his message of peace and non-violence fell on deaf ears.

My elders were respectful to Gandhiji, but up to a point. Some of my relatives were in the revolutionary parties, *Yugantar*, or *Anushilan*, which believed in armed struggle to fight the British. This was against Gandhiji's non-violent movement. Besides, being uprooted from their homes and habitat for generations, they were critical of Gandhiji for not being able to stop the partition of India. They had strong grievance, grouse, anguish, anger and *abhiman* (pride) about their losses. They could not forget and forgive that they lost everything, their livelihood, their home and hearth, their occupation and profession. Their women were raped and killed – at times in front of their own eyes. These curses of partition, for obvious reasons, were sometimes directed towards the Father of the Nation in particular and senior Congress and Muslim League leaders in general.

The point of anguish, as I have heard repeatedly, was that the leaders had not done enough to stop this massacre. Thus, the leader of leaders, Gandhiji, became the singled out person to be blamed by those aggrieved people. It was an emotional outburst.

Thousands of pages have been written about this in partition literature. Experts in history belonging to different camps wrote differently about the causes of partition. Many historians and commentators have written about the role played by British rulers during World War II. We all know about their dirty divide and rule policy. Tongues waggle even today about the friendship of the Mountbattens and Pandit Nehru. We know the role played by Muhammad Ali Jinnah and the Muslim League for the creation of Pakistan. All these stories have been widely documented by historians, journalists and commentators.

There is perhaps a non-biased history of our freedom struggle written by Dr. R. C. Mazumdar. He refused the offer of writing the history of India's struggle for Independence highlighting the singular role of the Congress Party. He wrote his own independent version, adding contributions made by revolutionaries, who believed in armed struggle and the Indian Naval Mutiny, 1946.

But the record of discussions, deliberations and negotiations conducted by our top political leaders on the one side, and the British team headed by the formidable Lord Mountbatten on the other, about the transition mechanisms from the British rule to India's freedom do not show our leaders in a sparkling color. They were certainly not tough negotiators. Besides, after Gandhiji declared the Quiet India movement on August 8, 1942, a large number of top and middle ranking leaders of the Congress as well other parties were arrested by the British rulers.

During this time of void, the British rulers hobnobbed with the idea of the partition. Muhammad Ali Jinnah and his Muslim League advocated the two-nation theory, i.e. two different independent states, one for the Hindus and the other for the Muslims, making a strong case for the creation of Pakistan as an independent state for the Muslims. Gurinder Chadha's BBC sponsored documentary (2017) on India's partition – an absorbing story – mentioned Jinnah's close contacts with Winston Churchill and others about this critical issue of dividing India[1]

It is also on record that some of our top leaders of the Congress Party stated that they were tired fighting for India's freedom and were eager to be rulers themselves soon. They were men in hurry.

The divide and rule policy of the British rulers was successful in dividing our political parties. The Muslim majority particularly in Bengal aspired to have their own State, Pakistan. Division of India became a historic reality, a kind of a fait accompli. While genuine experts, not the pseudo – or partisan experts, do know the detailed nuances of the complex history of partition, I am neither entering into this intellectual deliberation nor I am a historian. I am just narrating, to repeat, my own experience as a child from what people – the victims of the partition – used to perceive during those days.

I do intend to cover the people's perception as I have heard and experienced at a personal level. I am narrating the life story of the people who are victims of the partition. I am writing my story how I lived my life as a victim of partition. I have deep sorrow for losing my home. I have a strong emotional disconnect with the leaders who did not lose anything but gained a lot being rulers of Independent India. I have anger for suffering for no fault of mine. And I am not alone. Millions of people lost their homes, lost everything they possessed. They were on the run for their life.

Did our top leaders experience such miseries? They did not lose their home and hearth. Their wives and daughters were not assaulted or killed. They got more than enough return for their investment in the freedom struggle. They merrily walked over the dead bodies of the partition victims to their coveted throne of power. This was the perception of the people, I heard them talking animatedly. This is the real life history. This is the unwritten history.

Many of my close relatives and their friends joined the freedom movement, both non-violent as well as armed struggle, and were imprisoned under the British rule, lost their home, lost their youth. Even then, they were respectful to Gandhiji as a mass leader, who played a great role in making a huge number of Indians aware of the need for freedom. They could not accept the partition as a trophy of the Independence. Neither did Gandhiji.

Despite losing everything, they were happy at heart for the Independence of India. Unfortunately, those thousands who died could not celebrate the joy of living in a free country. Those alive accepted their poverty; they lived in free India with their pride. They do have a broader mind compared with that of their top leaders.

The Gandhian philosophy has many dimensions, not just politics alone. It showed a way of life, which is peaceful, and non-violent. The mode of protest – nay, a philosophy of life – is *Satyagraha* and *Ahimsa*, i.e., non-cooperation and non-violence.

Besides, Gandhiji did not run after power. He did not become President of the country. He never aspired for any position. He did fast on the day of Independence. He went on following his simple life. He wanted to disband the Congress Party, disband the military services after Independence. Whether his ideas were realistic or not was a different issue. He was on record to say this. He was honest in expressing his intentions. He gave his life, which was forcibly taken away by an assassin's bullet, leaving behind his direct disciples to enjoy power.

That is why my uncle, himself a freedom fighter, arranged this trip with many of us to see Gandhiji even for a glance. The truck was waiting at a particular spot in Beliaghata near a main road, which Gandhiji's entourage had to pass by. We waited for several hours. Then suddenly a covered jeep appeared and we vaguely heard *Ramdhoon* song from the slowly speeding jeep. People on the road shouted: Gandhiji *ki joy* (long live Gandhiji). Everybody said Gandhiji was in the jeep. This was my closest personal encounter with Gandhiji.

News of Gandhiji's assassination on January 30, 1948 was published in the special edition of newspapers. My father read the sad news and told the elders in the family. Next morning I saw my parents were cutting the full-page photograph of Gandhiji that was published in newspapers. They pasted the picture on a cardboard paper and placed it on a table in front of our entrance. A large garland of white flower was placed on the black and white photo of Gandhiji with huge quantity of loose flowers, all white. Incenses were burning, sweet smelling and bluish smoke was circling up. A multi-flame *dia* (lamp) was lit. It created quite an atmosphere.

In my father's mind the larger and holistic image of Gandhiji as a Mahatma was important, not the critical aspect of specific issues. He could fathom the significant leadership role of Gandhiji rather than blaming him for partition and its devastating human side, which dominated the minds of many affected people. Looking back my respect for my father rose immensely.

Throughout the day, literally hundreds of people came to pay their respect to Gandhiji. They brought in heaps of flowers. They went on discussing why such a great soul in a frail body was assassinated. Some people sat down and sang devotional songs. Some of my family members also joined.

I realized that something incredibly sad had happened, which should not have happened.

My Link with the Universe Snapped

It is an Air India flight, Boeing 747, the 'Queen of the Sky'. The 747 family has flown more than 5.6 billion people, equivalent to 80% of world population. I cannot sleep on the flight, at best doze off sometime. I also do not like movies on the small screen, though I see many passengers enjoy watching them. The earphone is a huge discomfort. Watching the slow movement of the flight map is very attractive to me. Besides, it is a wonderful time to contemplate.

Apparently, things were going fine. My younger brother Gobinda was born. I was going to school. I liked to go to school.

However, this small happiness was not to continue. My grandmother died one afternoon. Uprooted from her ancestral home in East Bengal, she was suffering internally. She was a dignified woman with a strong personality. She deeply felt sad about our predicament as a sequel to the partition. She used to sit silently by herself most of the time. She just died one afternoon. I heard later that it was a massive cerebral stroke.

My mother also fell ill. She was under the treatment of reputed Dr. Biren Bose, whose clinic was located on Russa Road, now rechristened as S.P. Mukherjee Road. As our makeshift residence did not have the required facilities, my mother was shifted to Chandannagar, about 35 kms from Calcutta. Chandannagar was a French colony since 1673; it was officially integrated with India on October 2, 1954. Jiban Bondhu uncle and his family were staying in a rented house there. It was a house with a garden and two *Shiva* temples standing near the front gate. On the other side, there was a sturdy two-storey building with large rooms. Rooms on the first floor had huge windows with strong iron rods from the floor level almost halfway up to the ceiling. In between there was a garden with many big trees and flower plants. It was a nice place. My mother was lying in the central room on the first floor; the room was very large. Day by day, she was getting worse. Within about a week of shifting to Chandannagar my mother breathed her last one afternoon.

I was thoroughly confused. I accompanied the body to the cremation *ghat* on the bank of the Hooghly River, popularly called, river Ganga and lit the pyre as was the Hindu practice, crying inconsolably. Somebody was holding my hand. How sad and devastated did a child feel in lighting his mother's pyre?

I sat down a little away from the funeral pyre of my mother's dead body. The glow of fire, the smell of burning human body, the flying fiery specs, the smell and crackling noise from the burning of wood and the human body sounded very cruel and horrific. My mother's flaming body was being reduced to ashes. The huge orange flame of the fire danced rhythmically, moved by the wind, smoke was spiraling up, and the spattering noise created a surrealistic and ghostly sight. The strong smoky smell of the burning human flesh permeated the air.

With a half and pale moon on the sky, the darkish grey water of the semi-circular shaped Ganga, making a soft and rolling sound, added a melancholic musical note to the whole sight.

I was looking at the dancing flame without blinking my eyes even though my eyes were burning. I was mesmerized. I just looked at the awesome sight and forgot everything else. My mother's body was engulfed by fire and was being reduced to ashes in front of my eyes. And I had to light the pyre! How cruel is the man who introduced this dreadful practice? Why do we have to follow such an unkind and inhuman practice of lighting the pyre on the face of the dead body of our near and dear ones? Why did I not protest? My mind was moving fast like a cinematic screen.

Looking at the clear, mid-night bluish sky, the vast and infinitely large mosaic of shinning stars and stars and stars, the floating clouds of ever changing shapes and sizes, I was thinking to which star my mother had gone to reside. When someone close dies, people say that the person resides there in one of the stars and looks at you, smiling and taking care of you from a distance. Amidst those countless stars, which one will be my mother's abode? Why had she to leave us and go so far in the sky to take care of us instead of living here with us?

Is it just a fairy tale? Is the not star a huge ball of fire, much bigger and hotter than the sun in our sky? How could anybody go there and reside? Why do our elders tell us such funny and wrong stories? They think they are consoling us. They think we are stupid kids. Adults may love us, but they certainly do not understand us.

In my tired and fatigued mind, these random thoughts were moving in a kaleidoscopic way. There were many questions coming and going in my mind in quick succession. But one particular question has been haunting me since then. It still does even today. Where does one actually go after death? Or is this the end of everything?

The fact is that she will not touch me again, hold me again, cuddle me again, and sing to me again. She just disappeared without even talking to me! My biological, emotional and spiritual links with the vast universe represented through my mother has just been snapped. I became alone, all alone amidst many people. I have permanently lost the biggest and most dependable pillar of love, affection and protection. This is the reality. I felt hopeless. At the same time, something was happening in my mind. My survival instinct was raising its head and giving a call. Take hold on yourself. You have to go a long way.

Some relatives were taking care of my father, who was profusely crying. Watching the burning pyre steadily, often looking at the clear sky with bright stars, the cool breeze from the river soothing my fatigued body, soft sound of the flowing water of the Ganga, all this made me to sleep off. Relatives forgot to take me home in their hurry.

They came back after several hours and found me unconscious. I went home leaving my mother on the bank of the river Ganga at Chandannagar.

The next day, in the evening, I was sitting with my sister near the large window of the first floor room where my mother was lying, I distinctly saw a lady in white sari, her head covered, softly asking me from the gate below: "Has your Suniti aunty come from Calcutta?" I said, "Yes" and asked her "to wait a moment. I am opening the gate".

I just turned my head to call somebody to open the front door. When I turned my head down towards her, she was gone!

I could not realize how a person who talked to me a couple seconds before could disappear in a moment. The road on both sides of the front door was a long straight line. To go in any direction will require at least a couple of minutes. All my relatives interpreted that the spirit of my mother came to check whether my aunt had come from Calcutta. When she heard that my aunt had come, she was relieved that Suniti aunt would take care of us.

However, I thought later that if she was a spirit, she could have realized that my aunt had already come. Then, why did she come clad in a white sari covering her fully and ask me about my aunt? It was too puzzling for me.

Ladies in the house stared talking together in loud voice, some started crying and yelling, some of them were blowing conch shells, it was a big hullaballoo. The spirit of my mother visited us! It's a grand occasion. I do not like such loud and crass high decibel expression of the so-called sorrow. Moments later, the same people would speak normally on some issues of material importance. Even as a child, I realized that their sorrow was not deep rooted. At the same time, they were not bad people.

Perhaps, that was normal. That was life! Would I also behave like them when I grow old? Someone from my inside told me, "just be what you are".

I felt very dizzy, mentally disturbed and went to the terrace, lay on my back looking at the evening sky. Stars were showing up one by one initially and then suddenly all appeared together. It looked just the same like the previous night. Which was the new star that my mother had become? Was it the one on the top right corner? Or the one on the left? I had to give up counting and mapping the night sky. The fact was that it looked marvelous. Looking at the cool and beautiful night sky, my mind got peace. I had to console myself that she must be there, one among the countless stars. I shut my eyes.

Surprisingly, images of my mother came to my mind. I opened my eyes to see if she was there. No, nobody was there. The same bluish sky with stars! I shut my eyes again. Thought of my mother, well she was back. Images of her followed me like a silent movie. She was fondling me, feeding me. Singing softly her favorite tune. Well, this was great! Whenever I wanted to see her, I would shut my eyes, and she was there. Even today, after almost seven long decades, when I think of her, remember her, want to see her, want to speak to her, I shut my eyes – and she is there, the same cool and composed face with a slight smile. I feel good.

My thought came back to the immediate incident. Was it a paranormal experience? What happened after death? Is not death an end of a person? Was there something called a soul as most people said? Were there ghosts? Was the woman in white a ghost of my mother? I was confused.

We came back to Kalighat. It took some time to settle down. Two persons – my grandmother and my mother, were gone. The size of the family was reduced. Relatives and friends came over to offer condolences. Everyone praised my mother. They expressed their personal experiences about my mother. I came to know a number of incidences of my mother's kindness and sweet behavior.

My friend Biren dropped in the afternoon; he tried to say some words of consolation, but could not go far, his eyes were misty. My friend Ranu from the neighborhood also turned up. She also could manage to mumble, "I am so sorry." She was in tears. When words failed to come out they held my hands softly, one each from one side, to transmit their feelings of love and empathy. When my childhood memory comes back to mind, I still feel the warmth of the two soft and warm palms that held my hand from two sides. I feel their presence. My childhood friends. They still live in my mind. After some time, Biren suggested, 'Let's play hide and seek'. We did play for some time. Smiles came back to our face. That was life, it moved on.

Surprisingly, our drill sir and the class teacher from my school also dropped in to express their sincere condolences. They spoke to my father and Suniti aunty. The drill sir hugged me. "Come to school tomorrow, son," he said. Class teacher Vinod sir took my hands. "See you tomorrow," he said with a warm smile. I felt assured. I was not alone.

Next evening my home tutor, Ramu da, came and told me in a matter of fact manner that he also lost his mother when he was five or six years old. He went on talking. We had no control on anybody's death. Now it was time to get back to work as the annual exam of first standard was nearing.

We got back to work. I completed my first standard exam with second rank. Life started moving on a low gear.

My father's illness was aggravating. There was no improvement. The shaking of the limbs seemed to have increased. Visits to Dr. B.C. Roy continued, albeit without any improvement.

Then yet another chapter of the tragic drama was unfolded. One afternoon I came from school and saw that our house was demolished. Everything was shattered into debris. I was shell-shocked. For the night, we got shelter under the staircase of the red building next door. The old man was kind, but tough at the same time. We will have to vacate his premises tomorrow before evening. I am homeless again.

My father had some friends who were top ranking politicians. They advised him to go to Sealdah station where refugees from East Bengal usually arrive by train. With great indignity suffered by my father, the next evening we shifted to Sealdah station premises where other refugee families were waiting to be the taken to the transit camp.

Goodbye, Biren. Goodbye, Ranu. Goodbye, drill sir. Goodbye, Vinod sir. Goodbye, Ramu da. They will be shocked to see the derbies of our house. They would be wondering what happened to us. Ramu da, drill sir, Vinod sir, Biren, Ranu – I will miss you all. Perhaps, I would not see them ever. I felt numb, thoughtless, and emotionless. Tears suddenly came from nowhere in steady streams. I did not try to wipe them dry. I held my sister and brother closely. They must not be lost in the crowd of Sealdah station.

Where are you Biren today? And Ranu? Both of you have also aged like me. Do you sometimes remember me?

CHAPTER 5

'Mushafir Bandho Gataria Bhudur Jana Hai'[1]

I look at the route map. The plane is still flying over the Atlantic. My back is paining – calf muscles are cramped. I take a walk around the cabin. A friendly flight attendant hands over a cup of coffee with a smiling face. We talk for a few minutes, 'cabbages and kings'. Back to my seat – mind moves to my childhood days.

Next morning we were taken by a truck to a transit camp; I guess, it was somewhere at Kashipur. We were treated like other refugees who had just arrived from East Bengal. We stayed side by side with many families on the first floor of a huge hall. It was very noisy. People shouting, quarrelling, trying to steal from others – it was a kind of living hell. The Government of West Bengal ran the transit camp, probably with the help of the Army. I saw many Army men around supervising works. We were served two meals of *khichari (a wholesome meal made of rice, pulses and some vegetables)* for lunch and dinner. We had to wait more than a week before they packed us off to Ranaghat Cooper's camp.

Five of us, my father, aunt, my sister, brother and I, had to stay in a tiny partitioned block under tin roof with thatched bamboo made walls.

My schooling stopped. Some former teachers, who were also there as refugees, started taking classes of Maths and English under the open sky. The camp administration helped to organize it. About 30 of us in different age groups were in one class. The classes ran for two hours. There was no book. They gave us some newsprint sheets and couple of pencils. Certain days, we went and came back as teachers were absent. Then one day we came to know that classes would not be held for an indefinite period as the teachers had opted for 'rehabilitation' and left. That was the end of school.

My father was very upset. His health was weak and his illness was aggravating. I was also not well. We survived on the free ration – certain quantity of inferior quality rice, pulses and some small amount of cash as dole. After a few months, my father enquired about the process of rehabilitation. About Rs. 5,000 and five *kathas*[2] of land would be given in some distant place. This meager amount of cash and a small piece of land was the so-called economic rehabilitation package for the refugees in West Bengal!

An agitation was building up among people who were compelled to leave their homes in East Bengal, run for safety and go to West Bengal. They lost their livelihood. They did not know any sophisticated professional skill. With only Rs. 5,000 and five *kathas* of land, how were they going to live?

Part of the money would be spent on frivolous consumption as they missed their normal food and lifestyle. The small amount of money would run out soon. How will they suddenly start a new profession? These were the questions. Besides, the easygoing lifestyle of Bengalis from East Bengal did not make them enterprising. In fact, it was not required for them to be enterprising.

People having leadership quality started organizing meetings where fiery speeches were delivered condemning politicians, particularly the Congress. The Left parties joined these agitations. In fact, the seeds of the growth of the Left parties were planted by the early 1950s. The refugee problem happened to be a great breeding ground for the left parties in West Bengal. There were protests, agitations, and rallies. Left parties, mainly the Communist Party of India, sided with the refugees. The refugees also thought that the opposition Left parties were their natural allies. They protested and criticized the Congress Governments in Delhi and West Bengal stating that Bengali refugees should not be sent outside Bengal. However, nobody listened to them.

The location for rehabilitation could be somewhere in West Bengal or Dandakaranya, a large and wide forest plateau area located in several Indian states such as Andhra Pradesh, Telengana, Chhattisgarh, Odisha and Maharashtra. The place is famous in the Ramayana where Ramachandra, Sita and Lakshmana went for their *vanavas* (penal exile).

Subsequently, Andaman Islands were also included as destinations for rehabilitation.

Selection of these two far off places for rehabilitation of Bengali refugees was received with hostility. People did not like to go to those places at all. Local people as well as administrations were not helpful and sympathetic. Eventually, finding no other alternatives, many refugees accepted their rehabilitation in both the remote places. Thousands of families ventured to take up these two destinations being desperate. Living in a refugee camp in such a shabby condition was unbearable. Nothing could be worse than this.

Incidentally, a large number of refugees from Dandakaranya were compelled to return to West Bengal in 1979. The Left Front Government, composed of the same leaders, who staunchly protested against the Congress Government's move to send Bengali refugees to Dandakaranya in earlier years, ironically changed their stand and forcefully deported back some 150,000 of them. However, some 40,000 refugees reached Marichjhapi in Sundarban areas and tried to settle there illegally. Marichjhapi is reserved as forestland. To move them out, the district administration tried to stop supply of food, drinking water and medicines! A court order stopped such inhuman action. Eventually, the Left Front Government ordered the police to evict them![3]

Besides refugee camps, there were colonies established by refugees on forcibly occupied land on outskirts and fringes of Calcutta. There were large number of such colonies named after leaders Netaji, Deshbandhu, Gandhiji, Bagha Jatin, et al. The colonies were also named after villages of East Bengal where from people had migrated.

Police and thugs of the land owners used to torture the refugees. There was discontentment all around. The original inhabitants of West Bengal did not obviously like this forcible intrusion. They certainly did not welcome refugees from the East. However, the refugees had nowhere to go. They had to survive somehow. They occupied the plots of land, unconcerned whether it was legal or illegal.

Suddenly, the population West Bengal, having a relatively small size of just 89 thousand sq kms, increased by over three million, immediately after partition. The flow continued even afterwards and the population density abruptly increased. Opportunities for education and employment were scarce. There was complete destabilization of everything in the State. I shall take up this in a later chapter.

Over the years, the illegal occupants were to be accepted. The colonies have now become well-settled localities. The Left Front Government took a bold initiative to hand over 99 year lease documents to residents of those colonies. Eventually, ownership documents were given to residents during the mid 2000s. Thus, after half a century residents of those colonies have become lawful owners. In fact, my sister-in-lawBratati, an officer of the concerned ministry, was closely involved in this task.

The original owners of the land had to suffer huge losses. They also suffered because of the partition.

My father was seriously thinking about rehabilitation. Though his health was failing, his mind was independent. He could not accept the condition of living in a refugee relief camp for an indefinitely long period. He decided to accept the offer of rehabilitation when it was announced that some limited number of plots were available at Simlagarh near Pandua, Hooghly district, about 65 kms from Calcutta, on the left side of GT Road. Though there was a rush for taking the offer, he with his persuasive power was able to convince officials.

We moved to Simlagarh, a sleepy village, largely unpopulated on the left side of the rail track and the GT Road. We stayed in tents for several months. Some amount of cash dole and food ration were provided for some weeks. A plot of land of five *kathas* was also allotted. My father made a modest mud walled house with two-sided slanting thatched roof. There were about 20 families with us in Simlagarh.

In the patch of land, my aunt started to grow certain types of vegetables. I helped her. We produced some quick growing vegetables for our consumption. There was a pond nearby. She made a fishing rod. She took me with her, showed me how to catch fish with a fishing line. Being a Brahmin widow if she touched fish she would have to take a bath. Some days I would spend long hours and was lucky to get some small fishes. That day the lunch and dinner became an occasion for celebration particularly for my sister and little brother! Tears used to flow from my aunts eyes. My father's eyes were also misty. They were thinking about the good days left behind.

About half a km away there was a huge banyan tree on the side of a big pond. The tree looked like a large umbrella. Many species of birds made it their home. They were always chirping and flying in and out.

One resident in this newly created colony was a former headmaster of a reputed school in East Bengal. He moved from house to house and collected about 15 children of various age groups. He made two divisions and started teaching. He also managed to get some books, slates, chalks, notebooks. After missing school for over one year, I was happy going to that class. For a couple of hours, I escaped the hardship of life. The teacher was very passionate about teaching. He was a teacher of English and Bengali literature. He could also teach arithmetic up to a level. He used to tell us stories from Shakespeare's *The Merchant of Venice, Julius Caesar, Macbeth*, Charles Dickens' *Oliver Twist, A Tell of Two Cities* besides reading Tagore's poems. His voice was deep and sweet, his recitation was very touching. I was very absorbed and tried to recite with him.

We used to go to Pandua, which was a historical site with several architectural structures. Pandua was also a market on both sides of GT Road. We bought all our essentials from Pandua. Sometimes I used to go to Pandua alone and visited the archaeological relics of the 13ᵗʰ century like the ruins of Pandu Raja's palace, the high raised minar, the mosque and Dargah built on the spot where Shah Safiuddin fell in a battle with one of the Pandu Rajas.

The story has it that cow slaughter was banned in Pandua. It was said that Shahid Shah Saifuddin, a young relative of Firozshah Khalji, the then Sultan of Delhi, was staying in Pandua for the circumcision ceremony of his son. Disregarding the King's order, he slaughtered a cow to serve beef to his guests. The angry King forcibly took Saifuddin's son and sacrificed the child to Goddess Kali!

When I was visiting Pandua as a kid, I did not know all this. Sitting on some of the relics, I used to shut my eyes and try to imagine how lively and colorful that place would have been hundreds of years ago!

Simlagarh used to be an island of peace and happiness temporarily. But the survival issue was related to earning, which was a big question then. My father was making trips to meet his friends in Calcutta in order to find something to do to earn a living. The dole given by the Government was running out.

Then something tragic happened. My brother Gobinda was not well at all. He looked very thin, could not eat much and suffered from occasional diarrhea. We took him to a doctor on the GT Road, close to Simlagarh station. He was treating Gobinda. One evening we had to take Gobinda to the doctor. He gave him a shot and some medicines. Those were the days of 'mixtures', which were made by the compounder attached to the doctor's clinic. Medical science was not as advanced as it was today.

Gobinda was on my aunt's arms. While we were returning home on foot, he developed spasms and breathing problem. We rushed back to the doctor. Gobinda was declared dead.

The doctor was very apologetic. My aunt argued with him. Heated words were exchanged. I smelled something wrong. I picked up the ampoule of the injection from the waste paper basket, which was given to Gobinda. People gathered around us. They also challenged the doctor. I heard that the wrong injection was given.

My father returned from Calcutta. One police officer with two constables also arrived and many neighbors were ready to help. The officer called the doctor. I told an uncle from the next door about the injection given by the doctor. I also told him about the conversation that took place at the clinic with the people around.

A meeting with the police officer, my father, some neighbors and the doctor began. Uncle took me to the meeting. He told the officer about the injection and handed him the ampoule. He mentioned that I picked it up. The officer thanked me for my alertness. They requested my father to forgive the doctor, who prostrated at the feet of my father and cried for the mistake. My father asked for some time to decide.

Yet another member of the family was gone forever! Until then, I held my tears for some time, but could not stop; it started flowing. I went out of the house, near the banyan tree, sat there and cried copiously.

Why are all these disastrous things happening to us?

More disasters were to follow. When I look back, I get a sad smile. In the following month during the early summer a storm with very strong wind and heavy rain, called *Kalbaishakhi*, the Nor'wester, had hit. Roofs of some houses including ours blew away. It rained heavily and we all got drenched. We took shelter in a neighbor's house, which survived the storm. I wondered why I too was not blown away.

My father was doing something during his frequent Calcutta trips. He managed to start a small shop to sell firewood in north Calcutta near Kumortuli, where idols such as Durga and other deities were made by the *patuas*, the idol makers.

The *patuas* are great artistes; they have been making beautiful idols generations after generations. Durga Puja is a magnificent and a colorful festival in West Bengal, thanks to the contributions of the *patuas* and all other artisans. Every year the idols are immersed after Puja is over. This gives the *patuas* an opportunity to add on to their imagination and skills for creating those magnificent and colorful idols. Equally, creative were the *pandol* makers, the decorators. The annual dismantling of their respective creations also gave them continuity in their livelihood, by providing an income every year. Thus, there is a continuity of artistic creativity as well as continuity of earning income. Indeed, a very pragmatic socio-economic model is in operation in West Bengal.

My father rented a small one-room accommodation. He also decided to send me to his elder sister Hemabala's family in Salkia, Howrah. My sister would stay with another family. The arrangement was temporary and meant for the renewal of our education. He was very worried about our education. He explained to me that there was no alternative. I could see that his eyes were misty. I knew he was a dignified and proud person. Because of ill health, he had become helpless. Both families welcomed us. Meanwhile, he would try hard to fight for survival, despite his weakening health.

CHAPTER

6

They Gave Me a Home, Loved and Took Care

*I was about to get up. Suddenly bumps, quite big ones, started. I sat down
somehow and put on the belt. I remember reading that bumps occur due to
turbulence. And Turbulence occurs due to the 'up and down motion of air the
plane is flying through.' It can sometime occur even in blue air condition – 'clear
air turbulence'. This is because the 'gravity wave' can even 'snake through clear
skies as easily through cloudy skies.'*[1] *It is not a bad idea to do some reading
before taking your first flight.*

I moved to Salkia, Howrah, on the other side of the river Ganga.
My aunt (eldest aunt) *Barapishi* and uncle Upendra Chakraborty,
Barapisho, as I was calling them, received me warmly. My uncle's elder
son Surendranath, *Barada*, second son Nripendranath, *Mejda*, the
youngest son Madhav, Madhu as he was called, and two sisters, my *Bardi*
and *Mejdi* were staying with their parents. Over and above, I joined
them. The sole earning member was my *Barada*, who was working as
an officer in a coal mining company. When I look back, my respect and
admiration for all of them reaches sky high.

I got admission in Salkia High School in the third standard. Madhu,
a few years older to me, was already there in fourth standard.

I was very happy and eagerly went to the school. *Mejda* was my
guardian in the school. I liked several teachers. One of them – Ganen
sir told us stories about his vacation trips all over India. He told us about
the vastness and diversity of our large country. He used to travel with an
economy budget. He said that he travelled living largely on bread and
banana, only rarely he would eat a vegetarian rice *thali*. He was a great
storyteller. He opened up the 'Incredible India' story to us.

I was coming within first to third rank in examinations. Once in a
half-yearly exam I came fourth. *Mejda* scolded me and visited the school

to meet the class teacher. The teacher assured him saying that difference in marks with the third was just one mark. He was so much concerned.

Mejda was an idiosyncratic person, with strong sense of personal dignity. He was studying diploma in electrical engineering, as the family could not afford the degree course because of expenses. He was a brilliant student in East Bengal. His academic and professional careers were disrupted by the partition. We all were de-classed, had to accept lesser education and lower positions in life.

He used to eat only rice, dal and one vegetable dish. He would never touch fish. He announced that he would eat fish only when he would start earning and contribute to support the family. A fantastic person!

Sometimes he would do electrical repair works in the neighborhood for a small earning. I was always with him as his assistant.

I enjoyed the love and affection of all. *Barda* was a difficult person, but he never complained that he had to support so many persons. He did not talk much to anybody in the house except me. He used to come home for lunch and had a short siesta. If I was at home, I had to wake him up at a particular time. Besides, during his siesta time I had to check whether he had grey hair; and pluck them, if they were there. But there hardly was any grey hair. He had nice black heavy locks of hair. That used to a be very difficult job. He treated his hair well by using Cantharidine perfumed hair oil, a popular brand in Bengal even today. He would not share it with anybody, and that is why he never kept it in the bathroom. Waking him by calling loudly, shaking his body and all that created a huge problem. Though my sisters did not like the harassment of mine, they were not in a position to say anything for obvious reasons.

One afternoon he was sleeping like a log. I could not wake him up. All in the family were watching with concern. I was very perturbed. Everybody in the house was standing there with worried face. When he eventually got up, he was late by more than an hour. He was angry and irritated and slapped me on the cheek. I was shocked, as nobody has ever hit me.

He soon understood that he should not have done this. However, my uncle was very upset and told *Barda* that he should never hit me again and stop this nonsense of waking him up. *Barda* left in hurry. Both my sisters consoled me. In the evening *Barda* came with large box of sweets, opened the box and offered me one, and asked me to distribute the sweets to all in the family. Sweets came to the house after a long time! I gave the first piece to my uncle, he took the sweet, shut his eyes and put his hand on my head and said some prayer. I felt happy and relaxed.

Late in the evening, I went to the terrace, sat down, and looked at the floating clouds in the moon lit sky. Tears started flowing from my eyes. I felt like a dependent, though not too badly cared for here, but certainly, it was not my home. Home need not be a palace. Neither need it be full of luxury, gourmet food, gorgeous dresses or many servants. Home is a home is a home, my own home, even if I have just two simple meals a day' and a plank to lie down.

There was no running water in the house. There was a municipal tap just outside our ground floor house on the road. Water used to be available for two hours in the morning and two hours in the evening. It was Madhu's and my job to collect the water in buckets and fill the drum inside the house. On both the rounds 20 buckets of water were required to be collected. Madhu used to take seven or eight; rest of it was on me to do. It was not an equal distribution, but I never complained. Madhu, in his own way, was protective of me in the school and outside. He was also my swimming coach. He was more experienced than Haran da. On holidays, both of us used to have our bath in a pond nearby. Madhu was an expert swimmer and he trained me to be a better swimmer. Because of Madhu, nobody could bully me in the school.

Both of us had to stand in the queue for drawing ration. There was a public distribution system those days. Rationed food grains like rice, wheat, pulses and sugar were supplied at reduced prices for fixed quantities allocated per person in the family. Usually food grains like rice were not available in the open market. These essential commodities were not usually available in the open market. Even if they were available, prices would be very high. Usually once a week, we had to stand in the queue for long hours. This ration was our life support system even though the food grains supplied were of inferior quality. Survival was the issue for the common man, not living.

I clearly remember certain experiences at Salkia. *Mejda* was a very strong sympathizer of the Communist Party. One night a senior leader came to stay for the night secretly. *Mejda* had taken permission from his father and *Barda*. They were all supporters of the party as it was siding with the refugees. *Mejda* brought some eggs and potatoes. A rich egg masala curry was prepared for all of us. Comrade leader (I never knew his name) arrived quietly at 10 O'clock at night. It was hush hush as the party, I heard, was banned those days. He took his dinner with just two items, dal and egg *masala* curry. He profusely praised the tasty food. He said, "My mother used to make very tasty food. I'm eating such good food after a long time."

He was a middle-aged person with very sober behavior. Easygoing and was talking to us all. He was a very friendly person without any ego.

At night, we used to sleep on the floor. Usually in the front room, hall in Bombay's parlance, *Barda,* uncle and Madhu used to sleep. In the large bedroom, we all used to sleep in three sets of beds spread on the floor. With mosquito nets of various shapes and sizes, it looked very messy. There was a kind of medium sized anteroom. One bed was made there for the guest, and a separate one for me. If he needed anything at night, I should help.

Before going to bed, comrade leader asked me many questions. He explained to me in a simple way so that I could understand who Karl Marx was, how he looked – with bushy hair and beard. He had a story telling style, repeating every now and then. He told me about Vladimir Ilyich Lenin. How he led the October Revolution in Russia in 1917. How the Communist Soviet Union was formed, dethroning the Tsarist regime of the Russia. He repeated what he thought would be difficult for me to understand. Do you get it? I nodded my head. Good, he continued. Everybody should get equal opportunity. A few persons must not acquire everything. Everybody should own everything. I understood some, but obviously missed a lot. My mind started thinking about these wonderful new ideas.

One day *Mejda* gave me a well-packed bundle of some books in a bag and told me to deliver the packet to my Upendra uncle's brother at his dentist's chamber in Sovabazar. He cautioned me repeatedly that I must not show the packet to anybody. I had visited the place once with *Mejda* and others. So one afternoon I had an adventure. I was given some coins for paying the fare for the ferryboat. I took the packet firmly in my hand, walked to Bandhaghat, Salkia on the shore of the river Ganga, took a steamer, crossed the river Ganga and landed on the other side. I walked up to the dentist's clinic on the first floor at the corner of Sovabazar Street.

I delivered the parcel to dentist uncle. He was surprised that I had come all alone. He escorted me back to the ferry stand. He waited until I walked up and the ferryboat started. I was touched by his affectionate concern. I repeated such trips a number of times.

Near our rented house in Salkia, there was a playground. Durga Puja, the gorgeous colorful weeklong festival of Bengalis, was organized there. I am talking about the early 1950s when the exuberant and pompous splendor of today's Durga Puja was not even dreamt of. Yet it was a very colorful festival with hearty and intimate inter-personal relations among the people of the community.

During the days of the Puja, gramophone records were played using an amplifier. For the first time I heard the popular play of Siraj ud-Daulah, the story of the last Nawab of Bengal, recorded on a gramophone disk. There was a big crowd raptly listening to the play. I was so moved when Miran, son of Mir Jafar, assassinated the young Nawab. Mir Jafar was the Commander-in-Chief of Siraj's 18,000 strong army. Besides, Siraj had the French allies with him. Mir Jafar had betrayed the Nawab by not joining the battle against the forces of the East India Company led by Col Robert Clive. Clive bribed Mir Jafar and promised that he would be made the next Nawab. They made a deal before the Battle of Plassey.

There were certain other powerful people including certain North-West Indian Marwari bankers like Jagat Seth, Omi Chand and Swarup Chand, who were settled in Bengal even those days. They sided with Mir Jafar and conspired against the Nawab at the instigation of Robert Clive. Clive's contingent was only 3,000. If the betrayal was not done, history would have been entirely different. Previously, Siraj had defeated the Company's forces and won over Calcutta, named it as Alinagar, and occupied Fort William in June 1756. However, this was a temporary victory.

The Battle of Plassey was lost within 40 minutes on June 23, 1757. Commander Mohanlal, Mir Madan and their small forces fought with vigor and became martyrs. But Siraj's large army, under the command of Mir Jafar, stood there motionless in a pathetic display of betrayal. With that defeat, the beginning of the Company Raj was launched in Bengal. The name Mir Jafar became synonymous with betrayer or conspirator.

Large numbers of people were standing near the megaphone, as we call it even today, listening to the play with watery eyes in rapt attention. The baritone voice of the person who voiced Siraj in the air mesmerized all of us. The play was very popular in Bengal. I used to listen to the play number of times, being fully absorbed. My eyes were also full of tears. I felt miserable because of the betrayal of Mir Jafar, and the palace politics and conspiracy of Ghaseti Begum, Siraj's maternal aunt. There was a dream sequence of Siraj, when he was emotionally saying to Aleya, the notch girl that '… I would again be the Nawab, I would sit on the throne; the prisoners would sing my praise…' Then Siraj was stabbed by Mir Jafar's son, Miran, shouting hoarsely; 'se sujog tomake dewa hobe na, Saitan' (you will not get that opportunity, Satan).

Even after so many years, I can still recite many of those lines. That was the beginning of the British rule, starting in Bengal, and then spreading across the whole country. When they left, they divided the country across religious lines, India and Pakistan.

My life has been connected with the historic defeat of Siraj!

Life moves on. While visiting my father and aunt in Nagerbazar, Dum Dum, a highly populated northern suburb of Calcutta, once on a vacation for a few days, I saw that in my father's cashbox – an old tin can of Lily Barley of those days – some Rs. 50 only were there. I counted and counted and counted; it was Rs. 50 only and not a rupee more. I was very sad and disturbed. Besides, I heard that my father and aunt had been living on some green vegetables and cheap, coarse rice only. I realized that my father's fuel wood shop was gone. With the help of a friend, he stared selling vegetables in the market! I was very sad and upset.

Next morning I joined my father in his vegetable selling endeavor totally against his will. His merchandise was a small number of cauliflowers. His friend came forward to meet me. Jatin uncle and his family also had to leave their home in East Bengal and come to West Bengal. They were also a reputed and well-off family. My father and Jatin uncle selling vegetables in a bazaar in Dum Dum was beyond my imagination. Still he was all smiles. "Do not take it bad, son. Every labor is honorable. We have to survive. I could not find anything else. I am managing somehow by doing this business," he said. He had a forced smile, trying to hide his tears. I touched his feet. Tears came to my eyes. He held me tight. He said, "We have to get past this. Go ahead with your education. When you all grow, get educated, all of us will be better off. Certain tough things do happen in life, which are beyond our control. Do not lose hope, son. You will do it." He patted my back several times and assured me.

He left in a huff, wiping his eyes. I sat on the small space allocated to us. I sold some cauliflowers in four hours, got over Rs. 50 with a profit of Rs. 20. For such a tiny scale of business, it was not bad. We could take care of that day's needs. In five days, we made a profit of over Rs. 100.

I discussed with my father to increase the volume of business by buying more cauliflower, but my father explained that the market's buying capacity was small. After we sold the last cauliflower, there was hardly any new customer. There were too many sellers and limited number of customers. If more cauliflowers were brought, there would be a large unsold stock – resulting in a loss. The unsold inventory would rot. I knew he had done his numbers. I got my first introduction to market economy.

My father told me that he would not do this for an indefinite period. He understood that something else would have to be done. His health deteriorated considerably. I could see that. I had to hide my tears. He assured me, "Go back to Salkia, finish your annual exam; this will take another two months. Thereafter we will stay together. Uma will also join us. Both of your educations will continue undisturbed."

He must have made some plans. Despite failing health, his fighting spirit was admirable. If he were physically all right, he would have taken care of us. He would have managed everything absolutely fine. He was capable. He was determined. He knew how to do business far better than many. But his health was deteriorating fast.

I looked at him and thought. This is my father Santosh Kumar Mukhopadhyay, tall and handsome even today, former treasurer of a Raj estate, used to living a comfortable life, taking care of several relatives, having an indomitable spirit, a fighting person despite deteriorating health, managing odds in life that had come aplenty, yet not succumbing to failure. My dear father! I love and respect you.

Tears, why do they come so often?

I passed my fourth standard annual exam with second rank. Meanwhile, my aunt Hemabala suddenly expired. My uncle's health also considerably deteriorated. My father came one day to take me back. He discussed with my uncle, *Barda* and others. I did not know where we were heading. I begged leave from all my present family members. Everybody's eyes were filled with tears. They all hugged me, blessed me. They gave me a home, took care of me with love and affection. I felt sad to leave them. My eyes were full of tears. They were wonderful people.

Destination Dhubulia Camp

The middle seat next to me is fortunately empty. An elderly woman is on the window seat; her head to toe wrapped with a blanket. A baby is crying hoarsely; its mother has been trying to pacify it. Lights are dim. Not unusual in long distance flight.

We came to Sealdah station and I was scared. My father told me not to be upset. He bought two tickets. We boarded Lalgola Express. Seeing me worried he said, "We were going to Dhubulia camp. It is not as crowded and unorganized like Ranaghat; it is spacious and well managed. Schools are there. I had no other alternative but to move over here. I tried my best to be on my own feet."

He continued, "My health is getting from bad to worse. The doctor told me that my movement would gradually become more difficult. You will be able to complete your school education here. And you won't have to stay with relatives howsoever good they are."

He also told me that he had surrendered the Simlagarh plot and had taken necessary permission for moving over to Dhubulia as there was no way to survive. The partition had run havoc in our lives, many, many lives…

During the British days Dhubulia, 112 kms from Calcutta, Nadia district, used to have a small airstrip, with a huge rectangular runway made of solid concrete. It was the base of the British Royal Air Force 99 Squadron from September to July 1944 and RAF 215 Squadron from December 28, 1944 until May 1, 1945. The mission of the RAF was to drop bombs on Japanese targets in Burma. It was also used for several other purposes.

We reached Dhubulia refugee camp after about four hours of journey. I understood that there really was no other alternative. I hoped that it would be better, somewhat more stable. And, I would be able to continue my schooling. Perhaps, a lower level equilibrium is better than complete disequilibrium.

We walked a long way from the Dhubulia railway station diagonally across fields to take a short cut. We reached our new home where my sister and Suniti aunt were already there. It was a small twin-room home with a smaller kitchen in the front. In one dwelling unit, four families were accommodated. Fortunately, ours was in one corner. Besides, there was a plot of land next to our block. Later on, we cultivated some quick growing seasonal vegetables on this plot of land.

After two years of separation from each other, we at last were united as a family – number reduced to four.

Next morning my father took me to school. It was a huge barrack with semi-circular tinned roof with solid brick walls on the sides, previously used by the Army and Air Force soldiers. The floor was smooth, cemented. On one side, there was a sort of a podium, a raised platform – the office. Thin dividers separated classes. I had to sit for a test. I had to write some Bengali and English words and was asked to write some sentences by one teacher. He was medium built, stout, wearing a half sleeved shirt and dhoti made of *Khadi* cotton. That meant he must be a Gandhian. The teacher liked my composition. I was admitted to standard fifth even without the Maths test. He of course carefully looked at my school reports and asked me a number of questions, some puzzling ones. Later I came to know that he was Sukumar sir, the Mathematics teacher.

The next day I went to school. I got some books, notebooks and pencils. There was no bench or table. Students had to bring their own mats to sit. It was a co-education school and the class teacher was Gayatri madam. A friendly person, she introduced me to the class of about 20 boys and girls. I got a warm reception.

I came to know that two new school buildings, one for boys and the other for girls, were under construction. We would move there in

January after our annual exam in December. We would be able to study up to 10ᵗʰ standard and appear for the school final examination.

We went to the Block 5 office of our area where my father already had us registered. I was introduced to the Ward Superintendent, Narayan Chandra Das. My father had already developed a mutually respectful relationship with him. He informed us that his family with children would also move over. His son would study here once the new school building was completed. Several other officials came to talk to me. We received our weekly dole of rice, wheat, dal and sugar. We also got some Australian saturated butter and milk powder. Over and above, we got certain amount of cash dole per head. Those were our fortnightly 'dole', in cash and kind from the Government. Besides, my father had a small amount of monthly pension from his former employer. We would have to survive on that. While going home I saw and felt bad about my father's misty eyes and subdued mood. I realized his sadness about living on Government doles. His ego, his proud personality was hurt. I held his hand. I did not say anything. It was neither necessary, nor possible. We swallowed our pride.

It was true that we got some relief. That would help us survive. My sister and I would be able to complete our schooling. In my mind, there was a painful feeling that the proud well-to-do family of ours would now live as refugees on food and cash doles from the Government. I was absolutely silent and trying to hold my tears. My father was a very sensitive and intelligent person. He understood my feeling.

He took me aside, held my hands and told me, "History has records of many refugee problems. Millions of people had to suffer; even die. World history is full with stories of refugee migration of people from one place to another." He continued, "You have seen that I tried my best to survive on my own. I tried several tiny businesses. I even sold vegetables. You also joined me for a week. You know it was very difficult to survive on such a petty and uncertain earning. My health has been steadily failing. If I am bedridden, what will happen to you all? I feel indignity in living on Government doles, but under the compelling circumstances, this is the only alternative. I am sure you will do the move over."

I realized. Later in the day, we went to meet the camp commander, Mr. Phanindra Bhusan Nag, popularly known as Phani Nag, a very tall and well-built person. He had a baritone voice. He could easily make a kid comfortable. He asked my name and in which class I was studying.

He told us "… two new school buildings will be ready within a few months, one for the boys and the other for the girls. I have already appointed several new teachers. There will be a good library, to be named after Chief Minister Dr. B.C. Roy's mother." He told me with a smile to drop in whenever I would like.

His office was in the middle of the camp, a small but sturdy and spacious building, which used to be the erstwhile British base commander's office. The new school and library buildings were under construction on the side on the National Highway No 34, connecting Calcutta with North Bengal. The market and other facilities, such as a dispensary, were also nearby. A doctor used to visit every morning. There was a large football field next to the dispensary.

On the other side of the railway line, there was the old camp, which started some years ago. There was a school already and a hospital, serving people of both old and new camps.

In December, we had our annual test. I came third in the class. That upset the previous pattern of the rank holders from third to first. They had to accept the new comer. Jhantu, Karunamoy, Kanan, Chameli and Rani, if I remember correctly, were in the toppers' list. I now joined them. So the competition became very stiff.

We moved to the new school building in January. The name of the school was Deshbandhu High School. It was affiliated to the Board of Secondary Education, West Bengal. It was box bracket shaped, with a large space for a garden in the front. The classrooms had new benches and tables. The girls school was named as Subash Chandra High School. Many teachers played an important role in our grooming.

In the initial years, there was Priyalal Das sir, a young and very enthusiastic teacher of the junior division. He was not very tall; but was strongly built with fair complexion, always with a smiling face. For some of us, he was our friend and mentor in the early years of our growing up. He played a significant role in our upbringing. He was closely involved with us for our extracurricular activities like athletics, football, bodybuilding and yoga exercises. He helped us to set up a club, Matri Mandir, and obtained a separate clubroom with an adjacent small playground for us, alongside an already existing club, Chatra Parishad. Mr. Nag was very cooperative and all this was done with his blessing.

Next to the school building, and on the side of the runway, there were teachers' quarters. Teachers with families were allotted one residential unit, somewhat better made than ours. Bachelor teachers or teachers who had not brought their families were given a room in a kind of row house; four/five rooms in a house.

Headmaster Annada Charan Bhowmick was a formidable personality, always in snow white *kurta* and *dhoti*. He used to teach English in senior classes, 9th and 10th standards. He had a baritone voice. Everyone was highly respectful to him. He had a great presence.

Among the other teachers from the junior classes, there also was Somshankar Sinha. He was tall and handsome, with a moderate stuttering voice. As I also had a bad stuttering and suffered from lack of confidence, he helped me with certain breathing and other exercises. He was a good painter. Along with Priyalal sir, he was closely involved in our club's literary and cultural activities. There were also Asit Sanyal and Billadas Banerjee, both of them too took great interest in our upbringing.

As a member of the club, we used to arrange several cultural functions, including yoga and bodybuilding shows. Football matches were organized. Priyalal sir along with a few other teachers used to organize a long walk to nearby villages. We used to have bath in the river *Jalangi,* flowing across the village Dhubulia, about two kilometers from our camp. It used to be great fun. We used to love Priyalal sir from our hearts.

Then one-day Priyalal sir announced that he would be leaving us to take a job in a school in Andaman Islands. It was a great shock for us. In his farewell function, many of us cried uncontrollably. He tried to soothe our feeling. Sir remains as an icon in my mind. When I write this homage to our 'Sir with Love', my eyes get misty.

Asit da was a teacher from the old camp's school, located on the other side of the railway station. He lived alone and as a great lover of flowers, he created a small garden in front of his quarters, which was full of many colorful flowers. What a great look it had! He had a love for driving road rollers. If one was found on the road, he would take the driver's seat and drive it for some time.

He was closely involved with us in the evenings in our club activities. He was interested in bodybuilding. He coached some senior students as well as some of us juniors. I enjoyed his affection a lot. He was a disciple of Mr. Universe, Monotosh Roy, a famous bodybuilder. I was very delighted. Monotosh Roy gave Asit da some advice about on how to train us.

After some months, in a cultural function, yoga, bodybuilding and athletics events were conducted with great fanfare. Those were thrilling days!

Then suddenly one day Asit da was also gone. He wrote me a letter after a couple of weeks saying how he would miss all of us and he was very sorry to leave us. He had to go because of some compulsions from his family and that he was in great hurry.

There was the Saraswati Puja day in the school and in our club. Balai da, a senior student was very creative. He used to make the idol with his own hands. We were his assistants. Balai da suffered a lot; he had tuberculosis. He was in the district hospital in Krishnanagar. We visited him in the hospital. He recovered within a few months. Soon his family opted for rehabilitation and left.

There was also Pijush da. He was a few years senior to us. He dropped out of school. He was engaged in business. He was like an elder brother to me, always very protective. He also ventured out and gone one day. Before going, he repeatedly told me that I must struggle hard and try moving up the ladder. He also arranged a feast for some of us before he left. He cooked chicken, and that was the first time I ate chicken curry with rice. Pijush da's cooking was heavenly.

As I was born in a Brahmin family, chicken was prohibited for us to eat. That was the orthodox custom. I have already mentioned that my mother used to make chicken soup for my father. It was possible only when we were living away from our family in Barisal.

Students deeply interested in theater would perform plays. I had no particular skill or talent in this area at all. It was a great joy to watch the historical plays like Siraj ud-Daulah, Chandra Gupta and Ashoka. The other club, Chatra Parishad, also organized theater shows. They also trained students to do a fantastic parade, military style, every Sunday morning.

Commercial *Yatra*, a folk theater performed on open stage with audiences all around. *Yatra* shows were usually very high-pitched and very melodramatic. It used to start late at night and end by early morning. I could never see full shows.

There were also seasonal performances of *Astra Prahra* (24 hours) *Hari Nam Sankirtan (Hare Krishna Hare Ram)* for one full fortnight 24x7 by a number of very famous groups from all over West Bengal. The composition, the tonal quality, and sounds of *mridangam or dhol* (drums on a sling hung from neck played by two palms) was of very high decibel. Some experts could play various musical tunes, including sounds such as running trains. People used to be glued to their performances the whole night.

There were football tournaments during monsoon season in the central football ground next to the market place. Inter-district competitions were also organized. Large number of people came to watch the matches. Two senior students using a megaphone gave running commentaries.

Many of us joined National Discipline Scheme (NDS), organized by the former soldiers of Netaji Subash Chandra Bose's Indian National Army (INA). This was before National Cadet Corps (NCC) was introduced at the degree college level. One of our instructors was Major Chandan Singh, who also fought in Netaji's INA. Like many, Major Singh was a great devotee of Netaji. He used to tell us many real life stories about Netaji and his forces' armed struggle against the British.

Under his rigorous training, we became strong, sturdy and disciplined. The standard of our parade improved considerably. We received full set of *khaki* uniforms. We felt great wearing the uniform and doing parades. Major Singh made us sweat a lot.

Nirmal, our classmate, was the group leader. He was tall, athletic and was very good in giving commands. He could have been a smart Army officer and would have surely risen high. Even I also started dreaming about a career in the Army.

Major Singh took the initiative of taking a battalion of us, composed of those selected to be the best, to Calcutta on the visit of Nikolai Bulganin, President of the Soviet Union and Nikita Khrushchev, Secretary General of the Communist Party in 1955 during their visit to India. We went to Calcutta to participate in a parade as a part of the celebration organized in their honor. But in the last minute, it was changed. Instead, we received an order to stand on one side of Jessore Road to welcome and wave at the moving cavalcade. Major Singh was very angry about the change of decision. However, he could not do anything as it was decided by the higher ups.

Though we felt let down, we were happy to be out of our routine life of Dhubulia. Being in Calcutta, watching the busy, colorful and high-speed life of the people, we really got enthused. We talked about it among ourselves, saying we would have to visit here later. We expressed our feelings to the Major and said that we were very thankful to him for arranging the trip.

Most probably, it was on India's Independence Day celebration, August 15 in 1957 that our school organized a big cultural function as well as a parade where Lt Col Jagannath Rao Bhosle, who was in Netaji's INA and also a Minister in Pandit Nehru's Government, was our chief guest. At the end, we sang the National Anthem. Our first attempt at singing the National Anthem did not please Lt Col Bhosle. I still remember Lt Col Bhosle's booming voice in praising the great valor and courage of Netaji Subash, the glorious fighting of the INA soldiers and asking us to be true inheritors of Netaji's ideals. As our first rendering of the National Anthem was too meek for him, he shouted from the dais to repeat it loudly. We did it a second time. He was not happy. We sang for the third time with our lungs out. "That's fine," he said, and continued, "When you sing the National Anthem, remember it is not just a song. Remember so many people gave up their lives struggling for the country's freedom. Your song must reach the sky so that they can hear that they are being remembered."

Those cultural performances, sports and games activities, made the life of residents not only bearable; they also helped, largely at least to elevate us from smaller and meaner issues. In a suddenly uprooted life, full of deprivations, agony, frustration, anger, mean and small-minded behavior were natural manifestations. Those cultural shows, sports and games as well the schooling of children diverted minds from harsh realities to somewhat higher levels. Those shows had an immense positive socio-psychological impact.

If those positive initiatives were not taken, life in a refugee camp would have been pathetic. Thousands and thousands of people suddenly uprooted from their age-old habitats were compelled to live in a cramped environment, huddling together. Most of them had nothing to do, while some enterprising people started some tiny shops like groceries in the neighborhood, or selling various merchandises in the market.

The deep sorrow of the refugees, the concern for the future of their children, the prospect of getting rehabilitated and moving out of the camp – all those issues made the people more sociable rather than becoming violent. The socio-cultural engagements helped immensely in making the society civil.

There were people from all districts of what was called East Bengal after partition. There were people from all cross sections of society. There were people from affluent class like those landed gentries, people from middle and low-income categories. There were people who were involved in farming, fishing, cattle rearing, people supplying every day needs like supply of milk, grocery, barbers, laundrymen, blacksmiths, cobblers, boatmen and such occupations, belonging to low and very low income earning groups. They all lived in Dhubulia camp doing nothing.

The abrupt uprooting created tensions, frustrations, anger and feeling of being deceived. In the cramped life lived on doles with not much hope of proper socio-economic rehabilitation sometimes there were outbursts, angry arguments on small issues, even violence. Such outbursts could have been much worse if Dhubulia did not get educational facilities cultural and sports activities around the year. Those activities had their therapeutic values in diverting minds of the frustrated people, without which life in the refugee camp would have been dehumanized.

Credit should go to authorities like camp commander Phani Nag and his team, school teachers and some leaders of the society. They managed the camp well and took great care of us. We would have rotted if they were not there when we were there.

CHAPTER

8

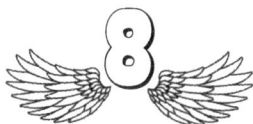

Growing Up Experiences

I am flying by Air India, the 'Palace in the Sky'. J R D Tata established Tata Air Services in 1932. He piloted the first-ever flight of the company from Karachi to Mumbai on October 15, 1932. The Government nationalized the company in 1953. JRD continued to be Chairman of Air India until 1978. Prime Minister Morarji Desai removed JRD without even informing him!

Our batch moved over to ninth standard, a turning point in our academic life. We had to appear in the school final exam, i.e. school leaving, in 1958–59. Our life would transcend to a possibly higher and a different level. Where should we go thereafter?

We were now senior students. We had a new group of teachers who not only taught us but also helped us in many ways. There was Arun Ghosh, teaching us Social Science, including limited portions of Economics as was in the syllabus, and History. He made a great impact on my mind. He walked with some difficulty due to an attack of polio when he was young. He always wore white dhoti and full-sleeved white shirt. I maintained a good relationship with him for long years. There was Santosh sir who taught us Civics and History. Both of their teaching styles and affectionate behavior made them dear to us. In fact, my love for Economics grew largely because of Arun Ghosh's teaching and off classroom interactions with him. Santosh sir made us realize the importance of History, without an objective perception of which our understanding of many things in societal life would be incomplete and unrealistic.

Sukumar sir taught us Maths. He used to give us a lot of homework, knowing well that nobody would be able to complete the task, say 20 sums to be done for the next day. He would check at random. No one would know whose turn would be the next. Even the same student might be asked to produce the task immediately on the subsequent day so that no one could take it easy. For the missed sum, the reward was one or two canings on the stretched out palm or a solid hit on the head by one or two fisted fingers, what in Bengali is known as *'gatta'*. In my generation, such treatment by caring teachers was common. We usually had no ill feeling about it. On the contrary, we were respectful to those teachers who took keen interest in the growing up of their students. The British public schools institutionalized such physical punishment. Today these are not acceptable.

There was Surendra Lal Maitra teaching us Science and Maths. Fair complexioned, bespectacled, yet with a sharply focused eye, tall, lean and thin, but with a glow of health, he was also an impact making teacher. He could make a difficult topic easy for us, a wonderful teacher. He took over as assistant headmaster later.

Over and above, there was the formidable head sir about whom I have already made mention. He lived without his family and on the weekend went home at Bali, near Calcutta, in Howrah district.

He took care of a stray dog. After an early lunch before the school, he would prepare a big ball of rice with some vegetables and fish, and feed the dog. The dog would in any case be waiting for his lunch.

Incidentally, it was, it still is, a practice in Bengal that before going to work people usually take an early lunch with some rice and a hot bowel of *dal*, some vegetables and fish curry. In those days, there was no cooking gas; cooking was done using coal as fuel. It took a long time to prepare the hearth. Smoke would belch out for a long time. The neighborhood would be polluted with thick and mushrooming smoke in the morning and evening. Besides, the practice was to go to market to buy fresh vegetables and fish every morning. By the time marketing was done, it would be time to go to office.

During lunchtime, the office-going people would eat some snacks. In downtown Calcutta, Dalhousie Square (BBD Bagh, as it is called now), a large number of mouth-watering street foods were available. The quality was reasonably good and price low. If you have watched Rick Stein's program on BBC on different cuisines in India, you might have noticed the huge varieties of food that was available on the streets of Calcutta's downtown. I did not miss an opportunity to have a grab when I was there during lunch time.

There was also Abani Taran Saha, teaching us Bengali. He was also an assistant headmaster. He himself was a well-known writer and poet. We became very close.

There were several other prominent teachers like Satish Bhattacharyay and Naresh Das, both teaching English and Ranjit Sarkar teaching History. Madhusudan Chakraborty was a good teacher, who later became a librarian. In various ways, these teachers took great care of us. We are very grateful to them; they went out of their way to help us. One of our English teachers, Bhupati sir, took the trouble of helping us with English grammar after 9 p.m., when everyone in his family had gone to bed. Some of us used to go to his house in the old camp area, more than one km from my home. We had to take a hurricane lantern for light to avoid snakes. He was doing this voluntarily. If we scored good marks he felt great and that was what he called his reward. Simple, at the same time, loving souls, many of them! We will not forget their love and affection.

Obviously, there were some bad ones too, whom we avoided.

The library, named after Chief Minister Dr. B.C. Roy's mother, Aghor Kamini Granthagar, became a great source of our learning. The new building, its fresh smell of paint, new books and magazines took us to the seventh heaven. The librarian, Madhusudan sir, was very helpful in guiding us to organize our reading habits.

I spent a lot of time in the library, reading various books. Like all in our class, I too was not very proficient in English. However, under the guidance of some of our teachers and the librarian, I made a journey unto this yet to be explored world. After some time, I was comfortable in getting the meaning out from books like *Oliver Twist, A Tell of Two Cities*, and *Around the World in Eighty Days*. I remember stories of some of these books from our classes under the banyan tree at Simlagarh.

On the day of the inauguration of the library, a colorful cultural function was organized. Dr. B.C. Roy, the Chief Minister of West Bengal, inaugurated the library named after his mother.

Apart from reading books from the library, some of us were very fond of reading Swapan Kumar's detective stories. These thin paperbacks had garishly colored covers. The price was a low, 50 *paise* per copy. Deepak Chatterjee was the hero, the detective, and his 'Watson' was Ratanlal. For us, it was a kind of daredevil story, where Deepak always solved the mystery. We also enjoyed descriptions like, 'the room is not too brightly lit, yet it is not too dark' and 'the road is not too wide, yet not too narrow'.

There was another detective story, which hit the stands later. The story had a woman detective. We read a couple of this series. Later we came across '*Dasshu Mohan*' stories. We liked them. We read Saradindu Bandopadhyaya's 'Boyamkesh' stories at a later stage in our life. We did not fall like a ton of bricks for Boyamkesh. He seemed too slow, lacked action packed thrills, a kind of a dhoti-shirt clad Bengali *Bhadralok* detective.

When we grew up and moved to the college, we became fond of H G Wells' *The Time Machine*, Arthur Conan Doyle's books, his characters Sherlock Holmes, his friend and assistant, Dr. Watson. Subsequently, many of us fell for Agatha Christie's crime fictions, her characters, Hercule Poirot and Miss Marple!

Some free days in the afternoon, my friend Ranjit and I used to visit Dulal da. He was a senior student with whom we became very friendly. He was very good in English but did not care for other subjects. He wanted to be out of school soon. Occasionally, we went to his house and then all three of us would walk a long distance along NH 34. Dulal da was an idiosyncratic person in many ways. He was always dressed in white dhoti, worn high over his ankle, and white shirt, either full or half-sleeved. He was fair complexioned and tall. He looked quite striking in white, drawing attention of many girls. But, he was not interested. He had a spiritual bent of mind, used to tell us about living a Spartan life, practicing yoga and meditation as well as celibacy. If he saw something 'bad', he would go out and look at the Sun for 'washing', nay 'purifying', his eyes! He was very good in playing the violin. We used to be often spellbound listening to him playing the violin. While playing a sad tune, which was his forte, tears would flow out from his eyes as well as ours.

He had two mothers, one his biological mother, *Bada* ma, and his father's second wife, his *Choto* ma. The two elderly women were staying in separate houses. They were widows, who had to live their lives under too many restrictions. I have already discussed this earlier.

Dulal da would eat at least two meals in a week at his *Choto* ma's place and rest with his biological mother, with whom he used to live. It might seem unlikely, but he was dear to both his mothers. We also enjoyed their affection. Dulal da's father died years ago. Actually, his father was killed at the time of riots. Talking about his father Dulal da could not control his emotion. He would cry like a child.

Dulal da left a strong impact on my mind. With time, we moved on to different paths of life. I lost contact with Dulal da after leaving Dhubulia. I heard that he lived his life as a sort of a monk somewhere in the northern suburbs of Calcutta.

Important people would be invited for our school functions. On one occasion Vivekananda Mukherjee, Chief Editor of *Yugantar Patrika,* a popular Bengali daily, was invited as chief guest. He was a well-known name in the country. With him came a popular Bengali litterateur, Abadhoot, who wrote the novel, later converted into a popular Bengali movie, *Maruthirtha Hinglas.* Abadhoot was his given name as a monk. He wore saffron colored clothes, as was the practice with Indian monks. He had an impressive figure and a strong personality. Ranjit and I were responsible for taking care of them. I was the editor of the hand-written school magazine. Abani sir introduced me to them as a budding author. I was very elated.

There was no teacher to teach Elective Mathematics, an important subject necessary to pursue education in Medical Science, Engineering or General Sciences. With Elective Mathematics, one could score very high marks unlike in literature or social sciences. A student had to choose an elective from a couple of subjects. It meant that whatever marks one gets out of 100, after deducting 30 from the marks scored by a student the balance marks would be added to his/her total marks. As such, I had to take Special Bengali as my elective subject, which was low scoring. Abani sir was of great help in teaching the subject.

Yet I was able to add 32 to my overall marks from all other compulsory subjects and was placed in the high first division. If I had elective mathematics, it would have been possible to add at least 55 to 60 marks to my total, which would have taken me to a much higher level of ranking.

As already discussed, the Communist Party stood by the problems of refugees. In our camp, several Communist Party leaders used to come to attend meetings. They delivered powerful and impact-making speeches in meetings organized by local leaders belonging to the committees formed for redressing grievances. The refugees became the natural support base of the Left parties in general and the Communist Party in particular.

The superintendent of our block allotted a separate room to me for studies. Opposite my study room, lived Kanai da, an up and coming Communist Party leader. He and his team used to invite many senior Communist Party leaders of high stature to visit Dhubulia and address meetings.

Comrade Renu Chakraborty, Member of Parliament, Comrade Mani Kuntala Sen, Member of Legislative Assembly, West Bengal, and Comrade Ambika Chakraborty of Chittagong armory attack fame were among many who addressed meetings organized by leaders of the refugee community.

On Kanai da's request, I gladly accommodated them in my so-called study for their night stay. The meetings used to go on until late in the evening, it was not possible for them to return to Calcutta. I was rather happy that they were spending the night in my room. This gave me an opportunity to talk to them, hear their experiences. They were also happy to talk to me. Despite being reputed leaders, they stayed in my humble room without any hassle. I preserved my autograph book, which also included their signatures, for long years.

There were some issues regarding books provided to us through grants given by the government. In fact, it used to be Central Government grants routed through the West Bengal Government. The school authorities informed us that no books would be provided to us when we reached 10th standard as the grants had been stopped. We were upset and protested. Local leaders also took up the issue and fought with the school and the camp authorities. Under the circumstances, some of us including me had to take a leadership role.

One afternoon Subhas Chakraborty, a student leader belonging to the students' wing of CPI based at Ranaghat, arrived. Later he became a powerful minister in the three and half decade long Left Front Government in West Bengal. He had a long conversation with us for understanding our problem. He had a very hefty diary where he wrote important points. He told me smilingly, "it is better to jot down the points, otherwise you may forget them". Mentally, I made a note. He was a smooth talker.

Eventually, a couple of local leaders from Communist Party, Krishnanagar took control of our agitation. On their advice, we organized a long procession from Dhubilia to Krishnanagar by road. It was distance of over 12 kilometers. About 30 of us walked a short distance on the National Highway 34 and then requested moving trucks to give us a lift. We had a nice ride and organized the procession again after reaching the destination.

Our leaders joined the procession from Krishnanagar. They went to the District Collector's office to discuss the issue and forward our memorandum. They came out of the meeting after half an hour and told us that everything would be all right. We should not worry. They left in a huff. They had not arranged even drinking water for us, not to speak of food. Certainly, we did not like the shabby treatment meted out to us.

Eventually, we got the books, perhaps on the merit of the case as was realized by the authorities. However, I am sure that there was a soft hand of our Head sir and camp commander Phani Nag in resolving the problem. Both of them were pursuing the case with their authorities. Some of us decided to go to Head sir and camp commander to offer apology and thanks. They received us warmly. They said that we should have depended on them. At the same time, they smilingly appreciated our organizational ability and leadership quality.

During this period, on Kanai da's initiative a few of us went to Calcutta with him one day to attend a huge meeting at the famous Calcutta Maidan in 1957 where the then Chinese Premier Zhou Enlai was the Chief Guest. Chief Minister Dr. B.C. Roy was also there on the dais. Even though what he spoke was not audible, we felt elated that we attended this large gathering and heard the voice of Zhou.

I came to know later that Zhou also came to India in 1954 to sign the *Pancha Sheel* (i.e, peaceful co-existence based on five moral principles like non – aggression, non-interference, equality and co-operation, etc.) treaty. He was also awarded a Honorary Doctorate degree by India International Peace Village during his visit in 1957.[1] Political relations between India and China were very good during those days. Slogans like *'Hindi Chini Bhai Bhai'* used to fill the air. Coming closer, these two great nations brought in a great hope for mutual co-operation in various areas. Pandit Nehru was influenced by the Chinese experiment of establishing an egalitarian society under the leadership of Mao Zedong. Nehru pleaded for American recognition of the Peoples Republic of China and its admission into the United Nations in the early 1950s.[2]

He was also influenced by the Soviet Russian system. He used the socialist approach of his own construct for developing the Indian economy in general and Indian industrial base in particular. But his hope was belied when China attacked India in 1962. Pandit Nehru suffered a bad shock; he died two years later in 1964.

CHAPTER

9

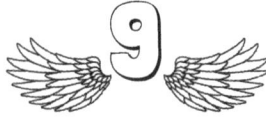

Phoenixes Have Risen

Indian passengers packed the flight. Many of them have been watching Hindi movies. You can meet a representative sample of the relatively well-off Indians on such a long distance flight. Over 25 million Indians travelled abroad in 2018 spending close to $ 20 billion compared with just three million in 1996. Both these numbers will have exponential growth in the near future.

We moved to 10th standard. We totally concentrated on our studies. Meanwhile, there were two significant developments. A job offer came for our senior batch that completed the school leaving examination. The Government of West Bengal introduced the State Transport Corporation, which would run buses in Calcutta. This was an initiative of Dr. B.C. Roy, the Chief Minister for refugee students. Many applied for the humble bus conductor's job. The salary was not high, but it was high enough to attract many. It was virtually a Government job, with full job security, benefits of provident fund and pension. Many of our senior friends joined as bus conductors. Some of them at least could have had a far better career. However, the marginal utility of money for those who do not have anything at all on hand would naturally be very high. For them some income today was better than higher income tomorrow. One had to live through today to see tomorrow.

This created some excitement in our community, including my family. Many of my friends, who could have a better career after completing graduation, did not wait for the uncertain future. The unhappiness was very intense when some of those who worked and earned better came home on holidays. My aunt was trying to give hints that I should accept the offer the following year. My father was against my joining it. He thought that if I accepted such a small job, my future would be sealed. I would be de-classed.

I remember Amalendu da, our senior. He could have got a top class career under normal circumstances. He was tall, well built, intelligent and good in studies. He was a good actor and good orator. In the historical plays, he used to don the role of Shah Jahan, the Mughal emperor. We used to be overawed by his presence. If he spoke to us, we would feel elated. But he had to take up the bus conductor's job as his family kept pressurizing him.

Years later one morning, I saw Amalendu da at the Garia bus depot. We came face to face. I looked at him somewhat puzzled. He smiled and called my name. He held my hands. "I know what you are thinking, Jiban. Take it easy. Tell me about you," he said. I told him that I just had a job as Economist in Tata Services, and would go to Mumbai soon. He hugged me and whispered, "Do not worry about me. I had no option. I wasted my life and career. I'm not unhappy. Tell me more about you. I think you are doing well."

We went for a cup of tea to a nearby rickety tea stall. Over the hot, thick and sweet tea, we chatted for a few minutes. He told me why he had to take up that job because of his family's massive emotional pressure. His parents expired a few years ago. He got married; they had a son, who was five years old. His wife was a teacher in a secondary school. He told me that they would ensure the boy's education, and give him full freedom in choosing his career. Amalendu da had organized his thoughts; he "dipped deep into his inside". He wished me well. I knew it came from his heart. We lost so many Amalendus because of the partition!

I thought of it. I decided that in the next year when such an offer would come, I would not accept it. I couldn't accept such a mundane job. I had to study further, complete my Masters and then make a career. I calculated that with the given cash and food doles, and my father's small pension from the estate, three persons could lead a normal life. My father told me, "Our life is finished; you must move on."

I always aspired to move up the ladder. Thinking about career options, though I did not have any clear idea about it. That was because

I had to choose an education, which should be inexpensive. I could not aspire to study medicine or engineering. Those would be expensive. That left me with two open areas, Humanities or Commerce. Yet I used to dream whether I would be able to reach the top slot. It may sound like daydreaming. However, I never ever gave up such day dreaming. At the same time, the curse of poverty was a brutal reality; it de-humanizes people. It had such a powerful gravity that it could crush a person's dream to a nightmarish dark hole.

The second development that happened was profoundly encouraging.

An apprentice monk, Bramachari Amar Chaitanya (Bishunu da as he was addressed) came to our school in 1958 with a small team from Ramakrishna Mission Ashram, Narendrapur, near Calcutta to interview students, who would be reaching ninth standard the following year for admission to their newly opened residential higher secondary school.

The school education system had radically been changed from the previous year to higher secondary system, meaning that school leaving would now be at 11th standard level, not 10th standard as it had been prevailing then.

A student had to decide whether he or she would opt for Fine Arts, Humanities, Commerce, Science or Technology. They would have to follow their chosen specialization and eventually make their careers accordingly. Thus, at a very early teen at about 14 years they would have to decide what career they would pursue. It would not be possible to change track thereafter. The system rigidity in India was ironical. That was ridiculous. Eventually, it was revised more or less to the old system in later years. Besides, curriculum at every level was also drastically revised and upgraded.

Our school also would follow the new pattern from the following year when the present eighth standard students would reach ninth standard. We were already in 10th standard; therefore, we had to follow the old system.

The monk from Ramakrishna Mission and his team conducted written and oral tests for academically good boys, who had completed their eighth standard. However, the opportunity was not open for girls. Schools run by Ramakrishna Mission all over India were boys' school.

Sarada Mission, the women's wing of the Ramakrishna order, ran the girls' school.

My friend Ranjit Mukherjee and a number of his batch mates appeared for the admission test. About eight students including Ranjit were selected. They would join the higher secondary school, a new residential school run by Ramakrishna Mission, Narendrapur soon. Bishnu da was the first headmaster of the school. The school started with many students from several refugee camps in 1958 and eventually became one of the best schools in the country. Bishnu da, later a renounced monk of Ramakrishna order, was none other than Swami Asaktananda.

Within less than a fortnight, Ranjit and my other friends left Dhubulia for Narendrapur, expecting a rosy future. All their expenses would be borne by grants from the Government. Students selected for studying at Ramakrishna Mission, Narendrapur School got a break in their lives and career. They were chosen from a number of refugee camps in West Bengal. Over a period, many students got such an opportunity.

Compared to those who took the job as bus conductors those selected students were luckier. Many of my friends Jadu, Nirmal, Paritosh and several others from senior classes took up the job as bus conductors. Each one of them could have had better career opportunities if their families had been a little more patient and allowed them to pursue their studies; or if they also aspired for better career options and were willing to run through the given difficult terrain for some more time.

I became alone. Ranjit and I were always moving together. The pressure of studies filled up that void. I had to go to Krishnanagar for appearing in the school final examination. I stayed with a family for four to five days when examinations were held every day. Every day there were two examinations, morning and afternoon. The host family was nice. They tried their best to make me as comfortable as possible. Then for the remaining examination days, I had to travel by train from Dhubulia to Krishnanagar. It was a distance of 12 kms. Sometimes trains were late, and as a result, there could be a problem of reaching the examination hall on time. Realizing that on two occasions, I went the previous evening and stayed the night with the helpful family. They were neither our relatives nor friends of our family. On somebody's request and recommendations, they accommodated me free of expenses. I was so grateful to their hospitality and care. Without their help, I would not have been able to appear for my school final examination. Who says there are no good souls on earth?

I successfully completed my school leaving with a high first division. That was the time to decide about the future. I came to know that students, if selected on merit, could study at Intermediate level and beyond staying at Ramakrishna Mission Ashram, Narendrapur. Ranjit helped me by sending application forms and necessary information.

The opportunity of college education was available for a smaller number of students of my time. Many of them, who were average in studies, eventually completed their school leaving and tried out smaller occupations like starting a small-scale business, largely retail trading. Their families got rehabilitation under various schemes in West Bengal, Dandakaranya or the Andaman Island as already mentioned. They had to settle down at a lower level of living standard. That option was somewhat better than staying in refugee camps.

Alongside the officially approved refugee rehabilitation centers, there were also large numbers of refugee colonies set up on illegally occupied lands. Areas adjacent to Calcutta like Jadavpur to Garia and beyond in the south were full of such colonies like Bijoygarh, Bagajatin, Netaji Nagar, Gandhi colony and many others. In the north, from Dum Dum to Barrackpore and on the Howrah main line, from Bali to Simlagarh had many pockets of such colonies.

People forcibly occupied colonies in all those areas, had to fight it out with the goons of the landlords. People stayed on, despite being beaten, and arrested, sometimes killed – they did not leave their plots. They organized themselves. It was a long drawn battle. Peaceful people living in East Bengal were forced to leave their homeland for generations, had to come to West Bengal and found that they were also not welcome there. They became desperate for survival.

When I am writing this piece, about 4.2 million people from Syria became displaced persons – refugees. They have been crossing the land route to European countries, many crossed the sea, many died, and those who reached the land found that they were not welcome. It was sad to see the photograph of the dead body of a well-dressed Syrian kid reaching the shores of Turkey. It hurt the conscience of the leaders of some West European countries. Germany and France welcomed the refugees on a quota system. Hungary, however, discouraged them by using cannon sprays and teargas shells. The border of Hungary and Serbia was shut. Cops with guns were waiting with fingers on triggers to shoot.

The destiny of refugees all over the world is the same, pathetic! The same is the destiny of refugees from East Pakistan who were forced to leave their home. Their survival instinct made them to forcibly occupy the land. By nature, they were peace loving, simple people. They had to fight to live, to save whatsoever family they had.

It took several years to settle down. The occupants organized themselves and elected committees to run their affairs. The committees took over the final distribution of plots of lands to families. Eventually, they made their poor men's home on those small plots of land. They started building schools, both for boys and girls.

The real life story of my freedom fighter father – in-law is the story of such desperate people. They all joined the freedom struggle when they were in schools or colleges. They gave up their youth for the sake of bringing freedom to India from the British Empire. They were arrested, sent to prison; some were served life or death sentence. My father-in-law, Taraprasad Chakraborty, was a leader of Anushilan Samiti, Dhaka from 1930 to 1946. Along with him there were 19 other freedom fighters including his younger brother Umaprasad. They all sacrificed their lives for the cause of the freedom of India. Taraprasad was a brilliant student. He plunged into the freedom movement after completing his school. He was imprisoned for 12 years. He did his graduation, postgraduation and graduation in law from the British prison. He studied Marxism in the prison. Many top rung Leftist leaders were his friends.

When he was out of the prison, it was time for the country to be free. However, the country would be divided into two on religious lines, India and Pakistan. Moreover, Pakistan would be divided into two segments, West and East. He was teaching in a college in Narayangung in 1946.

His family was living in Dhaka city. Their families also decided to move in batches. He took a small rented accommodation at Bhawanipur, South Calcutta. Then, along with some friends, he also moved to what is now Bijoygarh and got a small plot of land. He took the initiative to establish Bijoygarh Boys/Girls School as well as Bagha Jatin Girls School. He left active politics after partition. He took up a job in West Bengal Government. His children got their education there and life moved on. What a transition from an established family in the city of Dhaka to a small plot of land in an occupied area called Bijoygarh! There are thousands and thousands of such stories.

For example, a well to do family moved from Mymensingh District to a colony in Bijoygarh. The head of the family, Satish Ganguly (not real name), got a small plot. He had four children of different ages from a four-year to a 15-year-old. Except for the youngest, all others had been going to local schools, which were run by reasonably competent teachers found from the extended locality, or hired with a token salary. When the schools got official recognition, teachers and staff received their salary as per Government rules.

Abject poverty made the life of refugees miserable. The Ganguly family was no exception. Satish got a small job at a distant place wherefrom he could come home only on weekends. Satish's wife Aruna, once a beautiful person with a good personality, now reeling under the ravages of the bad time, managed to run the family in Satish's absence.

Usually, on Fridays both money and food stock would come down to the bottom. One Friday, Aruna went to the market and got just four heads of *hilsa* fish (the queen of fishes for the Bengali tongue) by paying just 50 *paise*! She had a small kitchen garden. She plucked a large-sized greenish colored *lau* (bottle gourd) and made a delicious preparation with it, mixed with the hilsa heads! *Loughanta* – delicious to the Bengali tongue.

Need for survival made them innovative. The locality was low lying with several ponds around. The water level of most ponds was almost up to the ground level. Sometimes kids would fall in the pond, drown and die. One such incident had happened. One day Aruna's youngest son went missing. She was alarmed and started shouting for her youngest boy. Finding him nowhere near the house, she was about to go out. But she realized the need to wear a blouse or petticoat, the necessary inner wear for the sari. She saw a *lungi* hanging, and tugged it, put it over the sari and ran, shouting the boy's name. When she found the boy at last, she thanked her Gods and Goddesses, and then gave a solid thrashing to the boy. The boy howled like hell for some time, then calmed down and went to sleep. In the evening everybody got some homemade, albeit mundane, sweet.

Under her strict and disciplined guidance, despite acute material deprivation, the next generation moved up. Two daughters were married well; their husbands prospered because of hard work. The eldest son became a qualified engineer, worked in the United States for many years. The youngest one obtained his civil engineering degree and became a wealthy developer/ builder. The second generation did even better. With her husband expired, Aruna lived alone in modest prosperity, supported by her children. The family had moved up to the next best level.

The women of the family had to take care of running the house as Aruna was doing. The male folks tried to earn some money by doing small jobs, managing small retail outlets, taking up some occupational activities like tailoring and teaching in schools, if educated. Surviving a day itself was an achievement. The bright students of higher standards like 9th or 10th would take tuitions to earn small additional income. Every small earning was of a great value. The marginal utility of the scarce money obviously was very high.

Usually the women knew how to run a kitchen garden. They started cultivating some easy growing vegetables like bottle gourd, bitter gourd, *ghinge* (ridge gourd), broad bean *or pue shank* (Ceylon spinach), the climbers which could grow on the roof; besides, bringal, raddish, spinach, lady's finger, chilis, which are small in size and shape and could grow on a small kitchen garden. Bottle gourds could grow in large numbers, if proper care was taken. Ladies knew, for example, that pouring water after washing rice, and the thick liquid that is available after boiling rice; both were good nutrients – free of cost organic fertilizers – for those vegetables. A dozen bottle gourds of various sizes could grow on a thatched roof. Besides, they also used to cultivate some easy growing regular and seasonal vegetables and flowers. That trait had come from their East Bengal heritage.

My mother-in-law used to do such gardening. Her coconut tree is a huge one today, producing a large numbers of fruits. I mentioned before how my aunt grew vegetables in the kitchen garden in Simlagarh and Dhubulia. I had also joined her in this endeavor. Such practice naturally came to them as a survival strategy.

Though somehow one or two daily meals could be arranged, clothes were extremely scarce. The lady of the house had just two old ordinary saris. Medicines were even more difficult to get because of high expenses. Many lived with their diseases. Who cared? Many died.

Over a period, the erstwhile forcibly occupied colonies were legalized. This took several decades. The small shabby dwelling units constructed by their fathers' generation had now been converted into much better brick and mortar buildings, sometime with imaginative designs.

There were thousands and thousands of such established dwelling units in Greater Calcutta areas like northern and southern suburbs. Walk through those colonies today, you would find them booming with life and activities. You would find the same if you travel across Howrah-Bardhaman main railway line. The same is the case if you travel from Sealdah station towards Barrackpore or Krishnanagar. Thanks to Calcutta Metropolitan Development Authority, these colonies have been provided with better roads, water, electricity and other basic amenities under the erstwhile Slum Improvement – not eradication – scheme of the CMPO. That was a unique and innovative urban development initiative.

Literally millions of people, uprooted because of partition, have somehow settled themselves in a very poor condition. The schools they set up initially with their own meager resources, eventually got approval from the Board of Secondary Education and the Government of West Bengal. Education for both boys and girls has helped students – my generation of young people – stand up in their strides, work intelligently hard and make a career. Their capital was education.

In earlier generations, girls' education was rare. Sister Nivedita (1867–1911) born out of Scottish-Irish parents was Swami Vivekananda's disciple. She had to go from door to door, begging parents for their girls to be admitted to her school, opened in November 1898, and had to shut the doors. If she were alive during the 1950s through 1960s, she would have been over joyous to see thousands and thousands of girls wearing uniforms and going to humble schools built by their partition-affected parents.

The school would start with devotional or patriotic songs and dedicated teachers taught them. From schools they would go to colleges, get their graduation and in many cases postgraduate degrees too. Backed by the educational qualification they were employed, started earning and took their lives to the next higher level. Their children both from those colonies as well as from refugee camps took the journey to the next higher level.

Literally, thousands passed out from those schools, many joined colleges for their graduation and few entered universities. The chain worked every year in increased numbers at every level. Then they took up jobs, joined some available occupations and stared making a living; improved their skills and reached higher levels. Life progressed in such a process.

They were young Phoenixes on the rise, spreading their wings in the Golden Sun. A quiet revolution was happening in Bengal.

Many belonging to the first generation of the partition-affected young people, largely speaking, the midnight's children did not get lost. They continuously tried hard and hard to move up higher echelons of society. Most of their parents had died by then. Their children constructed better buildings and well-furnished houses. They arranged better educational facilities for their children. Their creative initiatives, their challenge taking guts and their indomitable spirit generated a great dynamism in the socio-economic canvas of West Bengal.

At the same time, the deep anguish that they directly inherited from their parents made them sympathetic to Left ideologies.

Simultaneously, the art, culture, literature, painting crafts started flowing on, adding some color and shine to the subdued life. These are the success stories of my time, our time – the story of the royal Bengal tigers. It created a huge societal transformation and all that will be told as we go along. The disastrous effect of the partition was to some extent mitigated.

Meanwhile, at this juncture it must be briefly mentioned that the second generation of children, i.e. my son's generation, got much better educational opportunities – whether Engineering, Medicine, Commerce or Humanities – and moved up to next best rank – which is today's top rank. They got admissions to engineering and medical colleges or colleges providing education for Commerce and Humanities, depending on their merit. The budget provisioning for education in general and that for higher and technical education helped a lot, as the cost of such education was very low. Thus, they were able to take forward the baton of the relay race for living a life, not just surviving, to the next round.

Sometimes, either the elder son or daughter had to take the burden of running the family, take care of their old and diseased parents or elder relatives, educate their siblings, and so on and so forth. That put a heavy burden on their shoulders, sometimes crushing them.

When we watch Ritwik Ghatak's movies like *Meghe Dhaka Tara,* we see with deep sadness how the elder sister Neeta tried her best to take care of all in the family, including her elder brother who wanted to be a singer. Everybody in the family exploited her. Her old and diseased father loved her most but could not help her. When she got then incurable disease tuberculosis, how sadly she shouted, *Dada Ami Bachte Chai*! How will she live?

These sad and bitter real life stories, the stories of Neetas – the unsung heroines or heroes, of the epic of post partition Bengal – will find no place in history. Their contribution, their sacrifice helped their brothers and sisters to move forward in life and their parents to live on. However, the Neetas became expendable. Even beneficiaries might forget the benefactors. Life is cruel; well, if you leaf through Dark Nature[1], you would get what I am hinting at.

At the same time, many young persons could not move forward, either the circumstances were too hard for them or their motivation was not sufficient to take the stride. Some of them joined as foot soldiers of local political parties, or just wasted their lives. They chose their destiny, but they were in a minority.

Ramakrishna Mision Ashram, Narendrapur

"When everything seems to be against you, remember that an airplane takes-off against the wind, not with it.' – Henry Ford.

I applied for admission to study at intermediate level in Ramakrishna Mission Ashram, Narendrapur and received an interview letter. When I reached Narendrapur for the interview, I was impressed seeing the large and beautiful campus. I saw a number of my schoolmates from my school as well as the old camp school of Dhubulia, who had also applied.

After a couple of weeks, I received a postcard accepting my admission. I was thrilled. I explained to my father and aunt about the institute. They already knew some facts about the institute from Ranjit. Besides, my father was fully aware about the role and activities of Ramakrishna Mission and Math. The Math was a kind of monastery, while the Mission was usually a center of education, health or developmental activities.

When I was about to be admitted to Ramakrishna Mission Ashram, Narendrapur, my father reminded me about our short visit to Ramakrishna Math at Narayangung, Dhaka when I was a kid. He reminded me that the monk there had blessed me saying, '*Thakur tomar bhalo karun'* (Lord will bless you). He said and smiled, "Perhaps, this was what Thakur wished." He and my aunt were happy as my education would continue.

I reached Narendrapur one day in early June 1959 around 1 p.m. Ajit da, a young *Bramhachari* of Ramakrishna Math & Mission, received me in the office. The office was a simple tin shed, not like today's three-storey office building, which was built later. Ajit da was very tall, handsome and sweet-speaking young apprentice monk. He took me to Bramhananda Bhavan; a stone-colored three-storey dignified looking hostel building named after a direct disciple of Shree Ramakrishna. My room was on the front side of ground floor in one corner.

The building had a rectangular large garden on the front side. On the right, there was a pond. On the left and the rear, there was quite a longish S shaped lake. On the other side of the lake, four identical looking school hostels were located. Some more were constructed in later years. They were all similar in structure, the same zigzag shape and the same subdued yellow color. Only occupants were different with one building housing one particular batch of students.

While taking me first to the shrine on the first floor Ajit da asked me to do *pranam* to the decorated photographs of Shri Ramakrishna, Ma Sarada and Swami Vivekananda on the pedestal. He explained that every morning a bell would ring and everybody would have to assemble in the shrine to pray. The same would be in the evening. Prayer meant singing devotional songs, following a lead singer, largely composed for the Ramakrishna order and meditation. Then he took me to the dining hall, all the while explaining to me the schedule and all other things that I should know for living there and studying.

My first lunch in the hostel was served – rice, dal, one vegetable and fish curry. As I was late, the food was cold; it was bland in taste. Ajit da told me with twinkle in the eye that "when served hot, the food tastes better."

I came back to my room. Three students would stay in the room, each with a set of table and chair. There were three cupboards on the wall. I was more than happy about my room and furniture in it.

There were two large windows, one in the front, and the other on the right as I entered the room. There was a long corridor that I could see when the door was kept open. Since it was the lean season, not too many students were around. It was quiet. I looked through the right window. The main road of the campus passed through the *Aam Bagan* (Mango grove) and the new school building. The main office, auditorium and the college buildings were not there then. There was a playground in front of today's college building on one side, and the main office building on the other, next to the main gate.

On the left side from my window, I could see the tiny island on the lake with a small boat tied to a poll. There were a couple of wooden planks stretched from the main land to the island, a make shift bridge. It looked very tempting. Someday soon, I must go to the island and take a boat ride on the lake. The road from the main gate passed through a small concrete bridge to reach the other side of our hostel building. I felt at ease in mind. For the next two years, studying at intermediate level there would be no problem. Will see what would happen thereafter. I felt tired, and lay down on my bed and shut my eyes.

I wanted to study in Presidency College, but the authorities did not permit that. About 20 of our batch took admission at Intermediate level in the recently established Dinabandhu Andrews College, Garia, about three kilometers from Narendrapur. That was because of logistics. A bus would take all students in the morning and pick us back in the evening. Classes would start from the third week of June. We had about two weeks of free time.

There were a couple of weeks for the college to start. We were engaged in certain activities like cleaning the garden or moving furniture under the supervision of Ajit da. After a couple of hours of work, cold drinks were served, this was very refreshing. Besides, to inculcate in us the value of being respectful to any type of labor, we were paid Rs. 5 per day. In seven days, we earned Rs. 35 each. This work program helped all of us to know each other in our batch.

It was a great feeling for all of us who came from Dhubulia camp – we reached a place, which was not only beautiful but also congenial in every way. It was like a dream coming true. Within a short period, we were at home in Narendrapur.

Our college began. On the first day, we took a ride in the ashram bus, which dropped us near the college. The first day of college was nothing great.

The first class was on Bengali literature and the professor was a charmed speaker. He did not teach in the first class. Sitting atop the table, he told us stories, which we enjoyed. The next was the Logic class.

I realized that I would have to live with it somehow. The third class was on Accountancy, an otherwise damn boring subject, was taught superbly by the professor. He was impressively clad in snow-white dhoti and kurta. I liked that class.

Professor of English, Bina Madam, if I remember the name right; was a friendly person. She belonged to a well-known family of jewelers of Calcutta. Her informal and boisterous manners made her close to us.

There was another professor teaching English. Reserved and composed, she was meticulously dressed. She was teaching a rapid reader type of a book containing some interesting stories.

There was an engaging story of Eamon de Valera, the Irish freedom fighter, later the Head of the Government, and President of the Irish Republic. During the days of his freedom struggle, once he disguised himself as an old man who had to cross a river. There were many posters with the Eamon's photograph and reward of money for the person who would help cops to arrest Eamon. A young inspector was guarding the boats on the river, which Eamon, disguised as an old man, had to cross. The inspector was thinking that if he could catch the freedom fighter, the reward money would be helpful to his family. The old man was talking persuasively to the inspector. The inspector had a feeling that this old man was Eamon himself. Eventually, he allowed the old man to cross the river.

Our teacher – sorry, I forgot her name – was telling the story in such a dramatic way – as if enacting the episode – that when she finished, the whole class remained silent for a minute. It seemed that all of us were present there and were listening to the persuasive plea of the old man to the inspector. Then the class stood up and clapped. She smiled for the first time and thanked us.

As I did not study Elective Mathematics in 10th standard, I could not take the Science stream. That was a handicap. The option of studying Science was ruled out for me. I was admitted to Intermediate of Arts, i.e., Humanities stream. I was advised to take Economics, Logic and Accountancy along with two compulsory subjects English and Bengali literature. Besides, I would have to take another subject as an elective.

Over the weeks, we discussed among ourselves about what subject to take.

Eventually, some of us took a new, albeit non-academic, subject called Military Studies, with two papers. The first paper was theoretical and the second was to enroll in National Cadet Corps (NCC). The NCC was not compulsory then. As such, the facilities provided like uniform and food allowance were good and training camps were for long durations. Our NCC sir, a professor of Chemistry and holding a rank of a Major, was very competent instructor and friendly to us.

Two seniors studying Economics at Master's level became very friendly with me. One was Sagar da, who was a very bright student holding ranks in school leaving, intermediate and graduation levels. He used to recite poems of Rabindranath, Jibananada Das and others. His voice was booming. I became his instant disciple. The other was Rabi da, yet another very bright student. He was an examiner of our internal tests organized at the instance of Ranjan da, then a young *Bramhachari* of Ramakrishna order. He was the office supervisor and hostel warden. He kept an eye on our academics and arranged tests for various subjects. For the students of Humanities stream with Economics, he asked Rabi da to conduct the test. I scored high marks in Economics and that gave me good publicity. Thereafter I became close to him. I used to consult him on Economics subject related issues.

In our batch, there were about 12 students with a refugee background. We were given certain small jobs so that we could earn small amounts of pocket money. There was a bank in Narendrapur, which was not a full-fledged commercial bank. I heard that it was set up with the permission of the Reserve Bank of India. This small bank handled intra–ashram transactions. About four of us 'worked' in the bank on alternate evenings. I was assistant accountant, working under Ashu da, a senior student of engineering, who was the accountant. Ashu da, a bright student, was also an example of success. He also belonged to a partition-victim family. He made it great in his life and career.

My salary was Rs. 15 per month. The amount was not bad in those years. We used the money for personal expenses to buy the necessary daily items – toothpaste, soaps, laundry or for a haircut. The ashram authorities gave us our clothes and bedding – though the quality was inferior. I did not have a proper shoe for going to college. I had just one trouser. It was not bad; it served me a number of years. My father also made two visits to see where I was staying and studying. He was happy to see that I was in the right place.

Swami Lokeswasrananda, our *Bada Maharaj (head monk)*, was given the responsibility of running a students' home at Pathuriaghata, north Calcutta in his younger years. He gradually expanded the home. He selected many brilliant but poor students and helped them to complete their studies. Many of them eventually reached top positions in life and career in India or abroad. For running the establishment, he had to move from pillar to post to raise funds. Among his bright students, several also joined the Ramakrishna order as monks namely, Kalipada da, Ranjan da, Barun da, Bishnu da and Parameswer da.

Besides running the home, he also undertook social projects in neighboring slums of north Calcutta for helping poor people along with conducting night schools for illiterate adults as well as children. Students staying in the home used to render service in all those activities.

Bada Maharaj was a great organizer. He was very tall and handsome, soft spoken and with an aura around him. When I knew him better, I realized that he was a monk born much ahead of his time. He eventually became a father figure to me.

He thought of the problem of education in general and education of boys belonging to refugee families as well as other poor and unfortunate families. As such, he took the initiative to establish the Ramakrishna Mission Ashram, Narendrapur in 1956. Initially, it started with about 12 students from Pathuriaghata Home, north Calcutta, staying in tin sheds.

Lot of development had taken place during my stay of 13 years from 1959 to 1972. When I visited in later years, I found it unrecognizable. It had grown absolutely large with a huge campus in about 150 acres of lush green plot, with so many educational institutions from an autonomous university (as it is at present), a reputed secondary school, a well-run blind boys' academy, a technical institute, a large auditorium, a stadium to rural and agricultural training institutes and Lokashiksha Parishad.

All these institutions are located in picturesque surroundings of Narendrapur, erstwhile a small sleepy village close to Garia on one side and Sonarpur on the other. The school, the college, and the blind boys' school are top ranking institutions in the country.

The ashram has grown because of the wide vision as well as the organizational skill and leadership of Bada Maharaj. He built his team with then young monks as I have mentioned above. All of them eventually became leaders and successfully ran educational and social work institutions. When I went to Narendrapur in mid-1959, its expansion activities had just started.

During the two years of Intermediate level study, for me the most exciting experience was the two National Cadet Corps (NCC) camps, each for two weeks. We went to an old military establishment in Salua, 5 kms from IIT, Kharagpur on the State Highway 5. The Salua airstrip was an abandoned airbase used by the 317th Airlift Squadron of the US Air force during World War II. Presently Indian Air Force uses it as a Radar station. If I remember it correctly, we went for our NCC camp during 1959–61, twice or thrice for over two/ three weeks usually during summer vacation. About seven or eight of us were from Narendrapur.

The schedule was very hectic. The parade and many other sessions were very strict and tough. Even for a slight error, you got punished individually or as a team. You had to hold a rifle above your head, arms raised, and run around the large parade ground, twice or thrice. It was enough to take your heart out of your mouth

Swami Aksharananda, our Kalipada da, assistant secretary, Ramakrishna Mission, Narendrapur came to visit us in the camp one day. He was travelling with a couple of *Brahmacharis* and some senior students during the vacation. We were immensely happy to see that we were not alone and left out. We were happy that he loved us and so he took care of us; he took a long detour to visit us in the camp. The camp commander, our instructors and NCC sir were very happy to see the love and concern showed by Kalipada da, a monk of the Ramakrishna order.

In one of our camps, India's first ever Field Marshall Sam H.F.J. Manekshaw, when he was heading the Eastern Command, made a short visit to our camp. Our platoon was doing a vigorous parade for the selection of the best cadet. I was in the first row and one of the few cadets who shook hands with him. I was thrilled. Later in my life, I had a couple of occasions to meet him. He was the Director of a couple of Tata group companies – a fantastic person.

I still feel happy to remember that I was appointed Aide-de Camp (ADC) for a day to the camp commander (CC). I felt important to wear a beautiful shoulder band across my chest, walking a few steps ahead of the CC, with a baton under the arm. When you saw the ADC, you knew that the CC was around, and one would become alert. I enjoyed my one-day stint as ADC.

Apart from regular parades of very strenuous type, we were exposed to weapons handling, shooting and mock war. I realized that I could hit the bull's eye without much difficulty. My instructors were very impressed. My short-lived romance with military services, particularly Army began.

The ways of the human mind are fascinating – when you do meditation, you need to concentrate your mind. When you shoot a target, you need to concentrate your mind! One is to make your mind cool; the other is to kill!

Alongside, my aptitude for literary activities flourished. I already made some name as a poet when I was in school. I won several prizes. A teacher of mine from our school had taken my exercise book full of poems to a renowned literary figure, Ajit Chakraborty, who made appreciative comments. In the first two years in Narendrapur, I wrote many poems and short stories, which were published in reputed magazines and received appreciations and awards.

There was some contradiction in my personality, traits and aptitudes. Shyamal da, a senior student of English literature, who later became a monk of Ramakrishna order, used to say, "How come a poet can also be interested in the NCC!"

In public perception the image of a so-called Bengali poet was of someone not caring for himself, wearing shabby clothes, with beard and longish or bushy hair and a cloth bag hanging from his shoulder. It was not certainly the image of a powerful person – like a general in the Army.

We had to get up before dawn, have tea and go to the shrine for prayer. By 10 in the morning, we had an early lunch and were ready for the bus to take us to our college at Garia. On return, we got tea and snacks in the afternoon around 5 p.m. Prayer in the evening, was followed by study and dinner at around 9 p.m. We had to go with our plates for lunch and dinner. The lunch menu varied with a few changes on daily basis. Most days we would have rice, with dal, a vegetable and fish curry. Mutton and eggs were served one evening each week. Food was wholesome and hygienic. During festivals, the menu used to be gorgeous. It was like a food festival.

The food served in our Narendrapur ashram was non-vegetarian. There could be a perception that in Ramakrishna Mission food served would only be vegetarian. The fact is that in the vegetarian belt, the food served at Ramakrishna Math or Mission would be strictly vegetarian. In largely non-vegetarian locations, it usually is non-vegetarian.

On Sundays, our lunch was vegetarian, composed of a huge ball of boiled potato, with or without thinly sliced onions, a thick dal and a white and soft looking vegetable curry, with aesthetically cut potatoes, green bananas of a particular variety, sweet potatoes and beans in Bengali recipe known as *Sukto*. The taste was heavenly. The lunch ended with a tomato *chutney*, sweet in taste and curds.

Two of our friends could consume huge quantities of food. Those serving food got great joy in serving them. Many of us were onlookers encouraging them to gorge more food. Consuming three large balls of smashed potatoes along with more than double the quantity of all other items served required a super human capability. At times, we had to help them to stand!

There was lot of fun also in the hostel. There was no fan in our rooms. During summer nights, many went to the terrace to spread our beds and sleep under the open sky, sometimes starry and clear sky with a cool breeze. Some creative friends used to prepare specific designs about how to arrange the bedspreads each night. It could be flowery design, or like geometric patterns. I was not comfortable sleeping in the open. The terrace used to radiate heat at least for a few hours during early evening. One night I went up to see what the design was. I saw a great sight – heads were near the center and the bodies were like petals of a flower spread from the center! It was like a *'rangoli'* (colorful decoration on the floor) design. There were six such groups of sleeping beauties! If social media such as Facebook was active then, I am sure all the sleeping patterns would have created a riotous merriment to the world.

Two years of our Intermediate level education passed off smoothly. I successfully passed the Intermediate of Arts in first division. Then the question came: what next?

However, luck had it that the junior section (the initial formal name was Senior Basic School) of the school, standards six to eight, opened in 1961, with Parameswar da as headmaster.

Parameswar da was then a *Bramhachari*, who became Swami Umananda as a monk of the Ramakrishna order some years later. Over a period, he grew as one of the prominent leaders of the Ramakrishna Mission, successfully running activities of Ramakrishna Mission Branch, Purulia, an economically backward district of West Bengal, as secretary. Purulia Ramakrishna Mission also is a very reputed school. After obtaining monkhood, Parameswer da moved to Purulia as headmaster of the school, and later as secretary.

He invited me to teach in the junior school and move over to their hostel as a house master. I was more relieved than happy – it was a gift from the heavens.

The issue regarding my further studies was also solved as a residential degree college with only honors course had just opened in Narendrapur in 1960. If I studied in the new three-year degree college, I would have to study one extra year to graduate. The syllabuses of the three-year degree college with honors and masters levels for a subject like Economics had changed and upgraded significantly.

Some senior students including Sagar da and Rabi da advised me to go in for three-year degree course even though I would have to spend one extra year. Besides, expenses for education and living for students like me would be provided through funds largely coming from Refugee, Relief

& Rehabilitation Ministries, Governments of India and West Bengal as scholarship and, or stipend. I would not have to spend anything. Not only that, I would also be earning some income from teaching and other related activities. I would be able to send some money to my father every month.

I thought that it was the best, if not the only option for me. If I moved out from Narendrapur, I would have to earn for my education and living, which would be impossible to do. I promised to send more money every month to my father and aunt.

Thus, my immediate problem was solved. I moved over to the junior school hostel and started teaching several subjects like History, Geography and Social Studies. Simultaneously, I took admission to the three-year BA honors course in Ramakrishna Mission Residential College, Narendrapur, with Economics Honors as major (six papers of 100 marks each) and Political Science as subsidiary subject (300 marks). English and Bengali literature (150 marks each) were the two other compulsory subjects.

Many of my friends coming from similar background as of mine, expect a few, had to move out of the campus after the completion of our Intermediate level studies. Some of them joined whatsoever clerical or teaching jobs they could manage and continued with their graduate studies also. Those whose families had relatively better financial resources carried on with their studies. Others managed moving out and getting some small jobs as well as continuing their studies until graduation level.

At the same time, about eight students, including Ranjit, who all passed Intermediate level and/or higher secondary school with refugee camp background, were permitted to continue their stay in Narendrapur, took admission in the new degree course with different subjects as their honors. That would not have been possible if Ramakrishna Mission, Narendrapur would not have come forward to provide a helping hand to us.

There were many students like me with refugee background in the college. They all got their higher education and many of them joined various colleges and universities as professors. They moved up in the trajectory of life. Their children did better. I personally know many of them.

This happened because of the compassionate mind of Bada Maharaj; he helped all of us by giving a lifeline for our higher education and eventual career building. Without his help, we would not have made it.

When I think about it, I feel distressed for all those friends of mine in Dhubulia who took the easy and relatively poor option of taking up the job of bus conductor. Many of them were bright enough to qualify for entering the graduation course in our college.

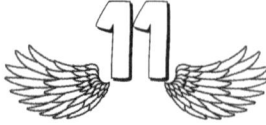

Building a Great Institution

J.R.D. Tata, the father of Indian aviation industry, wanted that when meals were served on flights, all lights must be on, windows open, the cutlery must sparkle! A food festival in the sky!

Ramakrishna Mission Ashram, Narendrapur is unique because a large number of educational institutions are built in a composite and picturesque campus. This vast complex has been systematically created under the overall guidance of Bada Maharaj.

As you enter from the main gate of Narendrapur, on the left is the new three-storey administrative office building, which was constructed in our presence. Join me for a quick tour. There is a large playground in front of the central office building and the college. The next building facing the gate was our four-storey college building with long corridors. Next to the college, on the left is the large auditorium, also constructed during our time. Thereafter is the higher secondary school building, facing which is the mango groove with a large number of trees in between an empty space. On the left end side of the garden, seats have been constructed. When I was teaching in the senior section, I took some of my classes here, getting comfortably soaked in the soft and silky winter sun. Students also enjoyed occasional outdoor classes.

Behind the school building is the technical institute where students, who have read up to 8th standard and staying in the neighborhood, were admitted for pursuing technical diploma. Ashrama authorities took care of the neighborhood community in several ways. Providing technical/ vocational education for boys was one of them.

Then there are rows of six school hostels across the lake, each looking similar though named separately after the direct disciples of Sri Ramakrishna. The road from the main gate takes the shape of a wide angled fork. The left one will take you to the guesthouse. The right one moves straight, with our college building, the auditorium and the school building on the left. After the school building, the road bends on the left and leads to the school hostels. In front of each hostel, there is a triangular shaped green garden with flowerbeds on the sides. The other arm of the road goes straight to Bramhananda Bhavan, the original 'home' where we students studying in outside colleges and universities used to stay. Morarji Desai, then Finance Minister of India, inaugurated the building in 1958. I stayed here during my first two years. It now houses college students.

At the turning point of the road is the Central Library, also constructed when we were there. Next to the library, stood the tall water tower, colored in Indian red with white on the top, which is now a landmark of the institute and visible from a long distance.

As you walk across the road, you could see flowerbeds in front of every building. During winter, colorful flowers and foliage would delight your mind. There was greenery all around with multi-colored flowerbeds, nurtured carefully, everywhere giving a look of paradise. On certain plots, seasonal vegetables were also grown.

Between the first two students' hostels is a road leading to the separate area of the Visually Challenged Boys' Academy, with the school building and hostels. This complex was built in the later years of my stay. In the beginning, visually challenged boys were staying in Bramhananda Bhavan. In fact, for some months I had a small visually challenged boy, Anup, as my roommate.

Bada Maharaj had a blind student, Bhabani Prasad Chanda, our Bhabani da, who was not only a bright student but also had leadership qualities. Bhabani da wrote to Bada Maharaj that he would like to study in a college and university but did not know how to go about it. Besides, he did not have resources. Bada Maharaj brought him to the home in north Calcutta where he stayed free of charge and studied up to Master's degree in History. Under the guidance of Bada Maharaj, Bhabani da started the Visually Challenged Boys' Academy, which became a great success. Shiba Prasad Sen Gupta, Shibu da, and Tarun da provided able assistance to Bhabani da. Both of them were qualified but visually challenged.

Presently, the academy has shifted to large garden house, the erstwhile Jethaika House, located between gate one and the main gate. The academy provides not only general education, but also training in computer operations, medical transcription, music and several vocational crafts to about 200 boys. There is also a Braille library and press. After the completion of the course, students are helped to get employment.

The road takes a circular turn and meets the other arm of the 'Y' shaped road across Bramhananda Bhavan. On the south of which is a pond where we bathed on some occasions during earlier years. On the further south side of the pond is Ramakrishnanda Bhavan, yet another longish three-storey school hostel where I stayed as house master for a couple of years. There is a new hostel building on the other side of the pond, where the original tin-shaded office building was located. Behind which is a narrow municipal road, followed by a large gym and a large playground where all major football, cricket and hockey matches were held. The construction of a stadium was about to be initiated when we were there, it has now been completed. Next to the present stadium, and on the side of the main road, there is a well-equipped gymnasium.

Swami Aksharananda, our Kalipada da, an ex-student of Bada Maharaj, was yet another stalwart. He was the assistant secretary of the ashram. He spent most of the working days of the week to get funding and grants form government and other institutional sources. He also supervised sports and games of the ashram along with Prasanta Da. Prasanta Giri was a professor of Statistics in our college. After the Independence of Bangladesh, Kalipada da became secretary of Dhaka branch of Ramakrishna Math & Mission. He travelled the length and breadth of that country and spread the secular message of Sri Ramakrishna's *Sarbadharma Samanayna* (unification of all religions). He became a much-respected person in Bangladesh too.

If you enter from gate number one, you can find a temple, which was not there at our time. On the right side of the temple, there is Lokashiksha Parishad office with classrooms and a museum of agricultural products. On the left of the road is the hostel for participants coming from rural and urban deprived areas to get training in agricultural extension work as well certain other income generating occupations.

The Parishad's activities cover, inter alia, 256 village organizations, five village development centers, several project offices and large number of cluster organizations spread across 12 districts of West Bengal. Activities of the Parishad include training and education in diverse vocational areas, agriculture and animal resource development programs, women and child development activities, health, hygiene and environmental awareness.

Since its inception in 1957 as the Institute of Social Education and Recreation, which was rechristened as the Lokashiksha Parishad in 1972, with widely expanded activities; thousands of people in hundreds of villages in West Bengal have been and are being helped to attain a higher standard of living.

After undergoing training here students could go back to their respective places and launch income generating or enhancing occupational activities. Trained supervisors from the Parishad go to sites and provide guidance periodically. As a result, their income shows a steady increase.

With great vision and foresight as well as profound love and affection Bada Maharaj created not only model educational institutes of national repute but also contributed greatly for rural development as well as urban slums. In this endeavor, he was helped by Barun da, Swami Prabhananda after attaining monkhood. Barun da was a brilliant student of Psychology, completed his master's degree with flying colors from the University of Calcutta. He was also a student of the north Calcutta home. Coming in close contact with Bada Maharaj, he eventually decided to renounce the material world and join the Ramakrishna order as a monk. He took the initiative of setting up what eventually became the Parishad. He also developed what was later known as Vivekananda Model of growth and development of rural areas through agriculture and allied activities for which the Parishad would provide training to concerned people of the locality with guidance and techniques. Recently, Swami Prabhananda was elevated as one of the three revered vice presidents of Ramakrishna Math and Mission, Belur Math.

Moving straight on the narrow road, you will find the poultry and a dairy farm, following which on the left side is the new monks' quarter, a small and Spartan ground-storey building. The original monks' quarter was also a tin-roofed shed.

During initial months of our inter-college study we had to take at least one course out of poultry, dairy, apiculture or sewing as a part of basic occupational activities based on Gandhiji's concept of basic education.

I opted for the poultry farming course. The head of both poultry and dairy farming was Ouderjyamoy Mitra, our Manik da. A trained singer of devotional songs, Manik da was also a very competent teacher. He was a hard taskmaster too.

One part of the poultry farm training, which we did not like at all, was the cleaning the birds enclaves. It smelled very bad. However, we had to do it; Manik da explained to us that unless cages of the birds were regularly cleaned, there could be infection, which might kill all birds.

One part of the training that we liked was picking eggs. It was great satisfaction to see birds laying eggs. When the egg lands gently on the ground; it is very soft and appears it might break. Soon the shell hardens and gradually takes its white color. Besides, it was wonderful to observe the satisfying expression of the mother hen.

The idea for undergoing such vocational education was that someday some of us might have to do such farming activities to support our income, or as a fall back option. The other point was that it would teach us value – that doing even a small and mundane work is respectable.

Actually, such training gave huge dividends to rural students of Lokshiksha Parishad. After undergoing various training courses, the students went back to their respective villages and were able to raise their income manifold. The agricultural extension/ training courses became, I heard later, a model of income generation programs in rural areas.

The management of the Parishad was taken over by Shuklaji from Barun da, who moved to take up other responsibilities. An old person with a silky silver mane on the head, and an ever-young mind, Shuklaji was a retired senior Indian Railway officer. He was medium sized, fair complexioned and always had a smile. We heard that he had a chance meeting with Bada Maharaj and decided thereafter to devote his time and energy to take over the activities of the Parishad.

Subsequently, Siba Prasad Chakraborty, Shibu da, a postgraduate in Social Works from TISS, was the person under whose leadership the activities of the Parishad reached great heights so much so that it attracted the attention of the World Bank. Even a Chinese delegation also visited several villages where the rural extension activities were going on under the guidance of the Parishad. He was also one of many students of Bada Maharaj who joined hands with him to make the dream successful. With his innovative approach and leadership skill, he was able to take the Parishad's activities to the next level.

In the later years, my friend Ranjit was very closely involved with the activities of the Parishad, which was very successful in raising the standard of living of the people in the project areas.

The road turns to the south, and then comes monks' dining hall – a spartan one – and a small, single-storey building where some ex-students like Pranab da, and Durga da, another ex-student and a professor of Philosophy of Calcutta University, and others including a former freedom fighter used to stay. On the other side of the stretched out road is the beautiful old bungalow with a fountain and large green space in front of the building, constructed by the Ispahani Group. M.M. Ispahani & Sons opened its office in Calcutta in 1900. After partition, they moved to Bangladesh. The Group is now a large business conglomerate in Bangladesh. They were the original owners of this part of the estate in Narendrapur.

The bungalow is now guesthouse for VIPs, many of whom visited our ashram regularly. Many eminent persons, ministers from Union and State Governments, leaders of various walks of society and guests, including foreigners visited our ashram. It was important to provide them with warm hospitality. I was there in the hospitality team. This helped me to develop lasting relationships with many of them.

As the road moves forward, there was a dance floor on the left, also made by the Ispahani Group. When we were on this side, we always came to the abandoned dance floor, stamped on the central area of the beautifully decorated floor, which was hollow and used to reverberate. It echoed the sound made from the floor.

Opposite to the dance hall was a large rectangular lake. It could have been good for boating. Across this lake is the newly constructed junior school building and three hostels, with a large ground in the middle with a large and old tree. There was a large playground behind the hostel on the left.

The road moves further and hits yet another narrow municipal road. Where the road took a bend before hitting the municipal road, there was the small office, the first ever office of the Institute of Social Education and Recreation (ISER) where Barun da, and then Shuklaji, used to sit and run the works of the Parishad during its first phase. On one side of the office of ISER was a beautiful, bushy *karamcha* tree, with a large circumference of dark green and somewhat thick leaves. It looked like a huge umbrella. During season, the abundance of blood red and snow white oval shaped *karamchas* would create a riot of colors. Seeing this beautiful tree, I went back to the memories of my dream house.

Crossing the municipal road, you enter the gate taking you to the central office and our college. Thus, the ashram land was in three large circular plots, connected by two municipal roads in between.

Kuber Maharaj, a senior monk, supervised the on-going construction projects inside our large campus. Besides, he oversaw projects like growing vegetables, fruits, flowers and gardening. Every day from 9 a.m. to 4 p.m., Kuber Maharaj personally supervised the projects spread across the 150-acre campus riding a paddled rickshaw. He also managed the cultivation of crops like paddy and certain pulses in the ashram's land outside the campus. He took care of the people who worked on these activities and maintained an affectionate relationship with the community outside the campus. He led an austere life and survived on one meal a day.

Establishing so many institutions in Narendrapur required superb vision, foresight and skill of a great inter-institutional leadership of very high caliber, which Bada Maharaj indeed possessed. Metaphorically, he was conducting a philharmonic orchestra like Zubin Mehta. It needed many players and leaders in each area. Bada Maharaj picked his team largely from his students as well as outsiders. Over a period, each one of them became leaders themselves and built precious institutions, and managed them competently.

Swami Vivekananda, the chief apostle of Shri Ramakrishna, established the Ramakrishna Math and Mission in 1899 at Belur, Howrah district of West Bengal, over an hour's drive from down town Calcutta. The motto of the Math & Mission is *Atmano mukshartham jagat hitayacha*", meaning, "For one's own salvation and the welfare of the world".[1]

To achieve this objective, our Bada Maharaj contributed his life, moving from setting up one institution to another. He devoted his full attention towards what Swami Vivekananda used to say, "man making by providing the right kind of education". The activities of various units of Narendrapur and their spillover effect in the outer society bear testimony to his dedicated and earnest endeavor. Students like us who had the privilege of getting our education under his overall guidance, those who provided services of all kinds from top level to the bottom, people who visited him would remember him as a loving and caring father figure. In the activities in which he spent his life, it could be said that he followed with full devotion the *jagat hitayacha*' part of the motto of Ramakrishna Math & Mission.

Alongside building institutions and successfully managing them, Bada Maharaj was himself an excellent orator and author. He spoke in a soft and sweet voice, in a story telling style. He could quickly touch listeners' minds. Actually, he was a 'spiritual ambassador' of India to many countries. He was also an author of repute. His books on Upanishads, for example, were so lucidly written that an average educated person could read and capture the meaning of these masterpieces.

It was a beautiful sight in the morning when Bada Maharaj would sit in his simple visiting room having tea and talking to people who would drop in for some work. He would be surrounded by all kinds of common birds including the ever-suspicious crows eating from his palm. There would also be dogs and cats as well to take their share of biscuits or puffed rice. He would touch and fondle the dogs and cats, while talking business with those people, who had come to see him with some purpose. This was a regular sight. I was in the audience on many occasions.

At the same time, as a monk he strenuously concentrated on the first part of the motto, '*atmana omokshartham*' as well. I may not be competent to say this, but I honestly feel that his spiritual attainment must have reached great heights. Even a short visit to him would make my mind cool and peaceful.

Narendrapur looks even more beautiful today. The trees and the greenery have grown in a healthy manner, making them look like a picture post card. The institutions within have also grown and expanded over the years.

Graduating Days

Couple of rows behind me a baby is crying; it is in high decibel – must be in serious discomfort. Changing air pressure could trouble them. Doctors advice to give something to babies to suck or swallow – to relieve the discomfort on flight. They could be cold; so proper warm clothes would help. 'Traveling with a toddler is like traveling with a rock band…' It requires careful planning and preparation.

Ramakrishna Mission Residential Degree College, Narendrapur was established in 1960, thanks to the huge organizational capability of Bikash da – a student of Bada Maharaj. Realizing his managerial talents, Bada Maharaj had chosen Bikash da to build the college. True to Bada Maharaj's conviction, Bikash da, who had just completed his Masters in Statistics, established the college in a record short time. Later in his life, Dr. Bikash C. Sanyal became a top UNESCO official.

The college was affiliated to the University of Calcutta. Initially, there were Physics, Chemistry, Mathematics and Statistics departments in the Science stream and Economics and English in the Humanities stream. Reputed teachers for all subjects from outside were invited to join as full time faculty members. A number of them were visiting professors. Physics and Chemistry labs were set up with latest equipment under the supervision of experts. The degree college gained autonomous status in 2008 and started postgraduate courses in Physics, Chemistry and English.

Our Economics department was on the fourth floor on the rear side. There were only seven students in our batch (1961–64), the second batch of the college. Teachers were largely senior ex-students. We had Prof. Rajen Chakraborty Thakur, Prof. Brajnandan Sinha and

Prof. Karunamoy Nandi, all senior students from Narendrapur. Prof. Debdas Chakraborty joined from outside. They all taught us with great care, though they were not experienced teachers. They were also easily accessible as they lived in the campus. The teacher-student ratio was high in our favor.

Besides, eminent faculty members in Economics from reputed colleges were also invited as visiting professors. Prof. Bhabatosh Dutta, a legendary Economics teacher from the Presidency College and Prof. Amlan Dutta, the eminent economist and thinker, from the University of Calcutta, were the two most respected teachers, who were invited to teach us. They helped us to open our horizon to various critical issues of Economics.

Prof. P.K. Roy was one visiting professor whom we cannot forget. He was always clad in white *dhoti* and k*urta* with the sleeves '*Geele Kara*' – creased fashionably. Bespectacled with gold-rimmed glasses, fair complexioned, handsome and very witty, he was fond of occasionally using *Bangal* dialect of the eastern part of Bengal.

He could teach all papers of Economics with equal ease and in a way, which would be very helpful for the university exam. Sometimes I used to arrange a good lunch for him in my school hostel. After enjoying an elaborate lunch, he would take sessions for four to five hours. His grip over subjects was very deep and delivery very pointed. He mixed his lectures with humor and wit, so his sessions used to be very absorbing. We are all very grateful to him.

Bikash da taught us a couple of topics in Statistics. He was very sharp and focused. Nanda Kishore De, Nanda da, yet another senior student, also taught Statistics. His style and method of teaching was simple and straightforward. He could make even an idiot understand the most difficult topics of the subject. There was also Prof. Prasanta Giri, Head of the Department of Statistics. He was yet another brilliant teacher. He could explain difficult problems in a very lucid and simple manner.

He was also in-charge of sports activities, though he did not play any games. Under Kalipada da's guidance, juniors Kartik da, Narayan da and Arun Das and Prasanta da used to run sports activities around the year. Football, hockey and cricket matches were regularly organized. Inter-district competitions were also organized. Every evening Bada Maharaj used to visit the ground to watch the matches, sometimes accompanied with some guests.

The ground used to be packed with students and outsiders. When a district-level football tournament was organized, people from neighboring areas came to watch matches. It was a good gesture as it helped, inter alia, to maintain good public relations. Expert players and coaches from reputed sports clubs of Calcutta trained students. Kartik da and Narayan da also played, while Arun was an excellent player; he used to play football, hockey and cricket. Besides, there was Haraprasad da, the stopper. Though I was not much of an athletic type, I played football in school. Finding no slot available in the football team, I took up hockey as a goalkeeper. I played for a couple of months in the first year. In one match, somebody accidentally hit me with a hockey stick on my chest and I fainted. That was the end of my career as a hockey player.

There is full-fledged stadium in the play ground.

Incidentally, this was also the time of newly introduced 'Nylon' synthetic fabric. Kartik da had a Nylon trouser. We all used to go to see and feel the soft fabric. Kartik da proudly told us, "You do not have to wash it frequently."

It was also the time when 'Hawai' *chappal* hit the Indian market. Many of us bought this new *chappal*. What we call Hawai *chappals* actually are flip-flops, popularized in the USA in the early 1960s as casual footwear. The history of flip-flops dates back to ancient Egyptians of 1500 BC. These were called thong sandals in ancient Greece. Even in ancient India, there is a wooden equivalent to sandals, known as *Kharam* with a toe-hold in the form of a raised knob, mostly worn by saints.

Today almost everybody in the world wears flips-flops. It became a craze in our time of the early 1960s. Many of us bought this *chappal*. But, some senior monks did not appreciate us wearing it. They thought that this *chappal* was an unnecessary luxury and at the same time useless.

Shantimoy Seal taught us Political Science. Though 'Pol Sc', in our shortcut vocabulary, was a subsidiary subject, he taught us with the seriousness of an honors subject. My hazy understanding of Marxism got some polish and streamlining under his teaching.

Being in an institution run by Ramakrishna Mission, we had to study Indian Culture, a subject structured by some senior monks. When introduced, students thought that it was an imposition. But later we felt grateful that it was introduced and as a result, we got familiar with the essence of the eternal message of Indian culture and heritage.

Ranjan da was elevated to monkhood as Swami Mumukshananda. Prior to this, he also completed his Masters of Philosophy examination with high marks as a private candidate. He became the first regular principal of our college. Subsequently he was posted as secretary, Ramakrishna Math, Mumbai branch, a posting that reflected his administrative capability. He also headed the Bramachari Training College, Belur Math. The objective of this unique 'college' was to provide the apprentice monks a sort of graduation course for two years so that they could be ideal monks of the Ramakrishna order. Along with administrative acumen, Ranjan da's scholastic talents and spiritual base were profound.

Incidentally, my memory was not bad at all. I could remember numbers of pages from prose, not to speak of poems, as well as numbers, like those of telephone or cars. I was like a telephone directory, providing service to many. This reminds me of one of our Intermediate level classmate whose memory was photographic. Sudip got five letter marks, i.e. 80% and above, in five subjects including Bengali literature & grammar at the school final exam. This was an astonishing performance. However, he got very low marks and failed in Mathematics. Therefore, he had to sit for a supplementary exam in Mathematics. He passed with very poor marks and joined us a couple of months late. He came from a rural area, which had no running water tap or electricity. He was amazed by turning the light switch on and off as well as the bathroom tap. What was amazing was that he could memorize several pages of any subject by just one quick reading. He could memorize and recite pages from Physics, Chemistry or Economics flawlessly. Unfortunately, his talent was not recognized. He failed in the Intermediate level final exam and disappeared.

Because of my part time teaching and other assignments in the junior section of the school, time was very short for my own studies. As house master of a junior school hostel, I had to perform certain tasks, which took a lot of time. I had to ensure that the boys got up before sunrise for prayer. I also introduced certain new systems. There were students' bodies and certain tasks allocated to some students. For example, one student was given an alarm clock and a bell for two weeks. He would move from one corner to the other from floor to floor ringing the bell. I revised the process. The bellhop would wake up one student each from one particular block of the hostel building, which had four blocks. Then a boy from each block would wake up one student from each room. It would be the duty of that boy from one room to wake up his roommates. During that time, the bell would continue to ring. That worked well and I changed the duty of students by rotation. I had to personally supervise the schedule every morning.

After the morning prayer, I had to see that everyone took part in the physical exercise. As I was NCC trained, I had to join the physical trainers more often than not. After tea, students had to go to the study hall. By turn, one house master had to be there to supervise and ensure that they studied. Some students would raise doubts about their subjects and the house master had to clear their doubts. The duration was one and half hours and I used to get the study hours duty one or two days in the morning.

As a result, my own study time was night hours. Quite often, I could not study at night due to fatigue. I had to earn some small amount of money, half of which I sent to my father and aunt. I had to manage my personal expenses with the other half. Certainly, I was not in a comfortable situation.

An all India inter-college literary contest on a specific theme of Swami Vivekananda's contributions was organized during the first year of my graduation. I won the first prize, which included a beautiful, large silver casket in the shape of a book and pen stand. It looked magnificent. There was a monetary component also, which I just signed in the books of accounts in the college office. Not a rupee was given to me.

The prize distribution was on the annual day held in the open mango grove. The function was presided over by Bada Maharaj. In the first year Dr. B.B. Mallik, Vice Chancellor, Calcutta University handed over the prize to me. I was flabbergasted with joy. There was no one close to share this joy. I won this first prize in the following two years too.

During those three years, I was student editor of our college magazine. If I remember it right, two issues were published. An edited and shorter version of my award-winning essay was published in the first one. In the second edition, I wrote a piece on Jesus Christ's so-called visit to India. It was known that there were a number of 'lost years' in Jesus' biographical documents. Nothing was mentioned about Jesus' life from 12 to 30 years of his age in the New Testament. My article was nothing original, it was based on the readings I did from some senior monks like Swami Abhedanandji, a brother disciple of Swami Vivekananda and a few others like reference to the Russian commentator, Nicolas Notovich, who wrote in 1887 that he found some writings regarding Jesus' stay and study in Hemis Monastery, presently in Ladakh. According to that version, Jesus came to India crossed Punjab, went to Puri, where he studied the esoteric Hindu literature. He went to Tibet. Swami Abhedanandaji himself visited Tibet and learned about that story. It became an interesting read because of the exciting nature of the topic. I heard later that Nicolas Notovich's story was investigated; it was found to be untrue.

Along with my tasks as house master and teacher in the junior school, I tried to widen the horizon of my knowledge by studying a number of books of various categories, including Literature, Political Science, History, Economic Development and biographies of eminent persons. In our degree course, we had to study the History of Economic Development of Russia, USA and Japan. I was very keenly following those classes, largely taken by Prof. Debdas Chakraborty. Those sessions helped me to understand nuances of various developmental paradigms. Besides, classes on Political Science by Prof. Seal provided me with the required philosophical and ideological settings. The follow-up readings beyond the course requirement helped me in my latter life. It helped me to widen my horizon.

Staying in the school student's hostel had certain additional benefits for a young person like me. One of them was to meet eminent persons whose children were studying there. I had opportunities to meet several Bengali novelists of repute and other celebrities. I was also able to develop a network with several correspondents and journalists from Calcutta-based newspapers.

The three years of our degree college education passed off more or less smoothly. The course had two terms, the first term examination was after the second year and the second term was at the end of third year. I successfully completed the course and got my BA honors degree in Economics. About 15 students with refugee background like me also successfully passed their honors graduation course in various subjects. We were able to achieve that because of opportunities provided by the Ramakrishna Mission, Narendrapur.

CHAPTER 13

Postgraduation and Beyond

I get up to take a walk. When I reach the rear, a young man gets up. He smiles and says, 'Recognize me, Sir?' I think fast, try to dig out his name, smile and say, "Surrender, right?" Both of us are happy to meet up in the sky. We exchange niceties, talk about our days in the Tata Group.

Though Jadavpur University was just about seven kms from Narendrapur, I decided to join the Department of Economics (DE), Calcutta University at Baranagar, on the other end of the city, about 35 kms. Due to inadequate road and rail transport facilities of mid-60s Calcutta, it used to take two hours each way. Almost everybody advised me not to be a fool. However, there were certain things fools would do which angels would never dare. I decided to become a fool. That was because in those days the rating of DE was the highest in the country.

DE included a galaxy of eminent teachers such as Dr. S.N. Sen, Prof. Amlan Dutta, Dr. Rakhal Dutta, Dr. Alak Ghosh, Dr. Amiya Baghchi, Dr. Nikhilesh Bhattacharyay, Dr. D.K. Basu, Dr. Santosh Bhattacharyay and part time teachers such as Dr. Ashok Mitra, Dr. Dhiresh Bhattacharyay, Prof. P.K. Roy and Dr. J.K. Sengupta. Many of those names were legends and noted scholars in the field of Economics teaching in Calcutta.

Dr. S.N.Sen, Head of the Department, took the very first class. He was a fatherly figure. He used to be invited as Chief Guest on certain occasions in Narendrapur such as the school's annual day. His wife always accompanied him. They were great admirers of Bada Maharaj. I used to render hospitality to them. His book *Central Banking in Underdeveloped Money Markets* was a very popular book. He eventually became Vice Chancellor of Calcutta University. He was also chairman of a commission set up by University Grants Commission. Dr. Sen Commission's recommendations for pay and perk increase, which were implemented all over India, made the life of college and university teachers not only comfortable but also respectable. It was my privilege to get the love and affection from Dr. Sen and his wife. I was also lucky to get in close contact with many eminent faculties and develop a cordial relationship with them.

For example, Prof. Amlan Dutta taught us Economic Thought and Philosophy in his inimitable logical flow. He was a highly erudite person with a strong rational bent of mind. As my attendance percentage fell short due to not being able to reach the department every day because of some assignment in the school or due to non – availability of transport, I had to take a number of tutorials under Prof. Dutta to make up for my absence in the class. My actual learning of Theoretical Economics started under his guidance. For this, I am profoundly grateful to him.

I realized the substantive thoroughness of Prof. Dutta's mind and intellect in later years. He later became Pro-Vice Chancellor, Finance of Calcutta University. He subsequently became Vice Chancellor of North Bengal University as well as Visva-Bharati University.

An author of over 20 books and papers both in Bengali and English on Economics and related isues; he was a prolific writer with a great style. Bertrand Russell wrote him a congratulatory note for authoring the book, '*For Democracy*', published in 1953 when he was just 29 years old.

In later years, I developed a close rapport with Prof. Dutta. When he visited Mumbai on certain occasions, he used to stay with me.

I took International Economics as my specialization paper. Prof. Roy taught some topics, and I liked his classes as I did in my graduation stage. He was a part time lecturer in the Department along with Dr. Dhiresh Bhattacharyay. Both of them were great teachers. In later years, I had an opportunity to work with Dr. Bhattacharyay for revising the Economics curriculum for higher secondary level. He was not only a wonderful teacher, but also a nice person.

I also admired Dr. Ashok Mitra, a versatile economist, intellectual, versatile author and commentator. His lectures were filled with bright sparks, sprinkled with wit, humor and sometimes cynicism.

He became the Finance Minister for several years of the Left Front Government in West Bengal headed by Jyoti Basu, which came to power in 1977 with a huge mandate. Dr. Mitra took up the issue of Central Government's deliberate negligence and step motherly treatment to West Bengal and the eastern region in a spirited way so much so that he used to be invited by several other states. In my early years with the Tata group, I remember that Mr. Somaiya, President of Indian Chamber of Commerce, Mumbai, invited him to give a talk on the subject. Mr. Somaiya introduced Dr. Mitra as his teacher in Harvard Business School with generous praise and admiration.

When I was in the second year in 1966, the Chinese Cultural Revolution had begun and the Vietnam War was still on. Hundreds of brilliant students had already joined the Naxalite movement. Posters used to appear on the walls of institutional buildings of Calcutta with stenciled print of Comrade Mao Zedong (pronounced then Mao Tse Tung) saying 'China's Chairman was Our Chairman'. All this created an impact in the young minds, particularly those wedded to Leftist ideology.

Dr. Mitra used to write a column, Calcutta Diary, in a new weekly, 'Now'. In fact, he wrote this column in several other magazines.[1] He wrote one piece about campus violence in 'Now' where he wrote about our batch, mentioning that he was coming to the campus, the Department of Economics to teach Economics. Usually bright students take up Economics. However, he did not find any sign of violence in our campus.

I had an occasion to meet him in India International Center, Delhi in 1971 when he was Chief Economic Adviser to Indira Gandhi's Government. He occupied many important positions in his career. But he was always in haste to quit. He had an elephant's memory and remembered that in the departments wall magazine, which I edited, there was a typo!

Dr. J.K. Sengupta, yet another brilliant teacher, specializing in Operation Research, came back from the States to teach in IIM-C in Calcutta, where he became Director. He used to take sessions on Growth Theories. His lecture was highly Mathematics oriented; the black board would be full of equations. He often took three to four sessions at a stretch. When he spoke, we became spell bound, not that we understood much. We took hurried notes and improved the content by consulting among ourselves. Reading those topics later would reveal the meaning to us.

Bikash da invited him to our college in Narendrapur. I had to take care of minute details of his visit and that gave me an opportunity to know him better. I spent almost one full day with him. He spoke to me on Economics related issues and asked me questions about India as well as West Bengal, which I tried to answer. He also asked some personal questions. At the end, he advised me to do research work.

There were about 20 girl students in our batch of about 120 students. In those days, girls had to sit separately on one side, close to the teacher's platform. Some of them belonged to orthodox families. A couple of them would enter the class along with the teacher. The practice of segregating boys and girls was not in vogue in the mid 1960s.

There were groups among students like, the Presidency group or St Xavier's group based on which college they studied. There were five students from Narendrapur college. Ours was a new college and many even did not know about it. However, over time, we mingled across territorial lines and became good friends.

The Left minded student group of our batch formed the autonomous students union, defeating the Chatra Parishad of the Congress. Three of us from Narendrapur became office bearers. Amitava was elected general secretary, Kanak Debating Society and I became the Magazine Editor. Once in a lighter vein, Dr. Sen told Bada Maharaj in my presence, "… Your students are all Left oriented."

There were several other brilliant students in our batch. It used to be great to interact with them. Many of them reached great heights in their respective fields like banking, government services, education, corporate sector or politics. For example, Dr. Asim Das Gupta became Finance Minister of the Left Front Government for almost a quarter century until 2011. People in the respective fields appreciated his contributions to the country's indirect tax reforms like VAT and GST. Students admired him as a very competent teacher.

I also taught in the junior school in Narendrapur when doing my Masters, took care of the hostel as house master and ran the school library. The tasks helped me earn Rs. 300 per month, half of which I sent to my father and aunt. My boarding and lodging were taken care of by the school. I had to manage my personal expenses with about Rs. 150. Books were available in the college library. I had to work for my and my family's survival. The result again was lack of time for my studies.

Many of my batch mates were staying in the hostel in single rooms adjacent to the department. They could afford the expenses as they belonged to relatively well-off families. Some of my friends used to conduct private tuitions to cover their pocket expenses, over and above the financial support they received from their parents. I thought staying in Narendrapur was the best option for completing my education. I had to squeeze in time for my studies.

During this time, Parameswer da wanted me to give a talk on India's five-year plan to students and teachers. I was quite scared because of my stuttering. I told myself that I do teach in classes and manage my class fine. Therefore, that would also be fine. Yet there was tension. If I were conscious about it, I would stutter. It is easy to talk, but difficult to perform. Yet, I decided to go ahead. I organized my speech in a simple way so that our junior school students could understand the evolution of our planning process from the first plan to the fourth plan. Some teachers were also there. To my surprise, it went off well. Parameswer da congratulated me. "I knew, Jiban, you will do it," he said. My friends also told me that I explained the nuances of the plans and details in a simple way. It was effective communication. Students saw me in a new role and I was relaxed.

My confidence grew. Looking back, I realized that had Parameswer da not pushed me, I might not have got out of the problem.

Hearing that he was not well, I went to visit him recently in the senior monks' home in Belur Math. He was old and not too well physically, but he had that serene smile on his face. He was very happy to see me. We talked about our days in Narendrapur. I reminded him about how he made me a teacher and pushed me to give a public talk. He smiled and patted my back. I had tears in my eyes. His whole life, full of vibrant enthusiasm and service rendering activities, came to me like a flash back. As a monk he was so positively active and, at the same time, very composed. Old age does not spare anybody, not even a monk.

Because of the unrest in the campus, our MA exam got postponed to early 1967. In our center of examination, the law college building in Ballygangue, there was violence in some classrooms on certain days. Students in those classrooms were not allowed to write the exam of one paper. Goons tore our answer papers and threw them out. I was in one such classroom. The goons forcibly took my answer paper and threw it out of the window. As a result, some of us had to rewrite that paper after about three months.

Immediately after our MA exam, the written test for the newly introduced Indian Economics Service (IES) was held. I appeared for the first two days. However, the Governor of West Bengal dismissed the United Front (UF) Government at the instance of the Central Government. The dislodged UF immediately announced two full days of *bandh*. I could not reach the exam center for the third day's examination.

Political parties never bother to consider that thousands of common people are adversely affected because of a sudden call for a total *bandh*. *Bandhs*, agitation, lengthy processions are part of life in Calcutta even today, announced by every political party.

Understandably, processions, protest meetings and strikes are means of taking up issues in a democracy against harmful decisions of the sitting Government or establishments. However, when they are announced habitually or randomly, they disrupt the normal life of people at large.

When the result came for my incomplete written test, I was both happy and sad at the same time. I got very high marks but missed the opportunity. If I had been able to appear for the last day's test, I would have certainly qualified for the oral interview.

Later in my career, I had the opportunity to meet some first batch IES officers working on lien with IDBI, Mumbai. They were very unhappy about their job. In fact, both IES and ISS (Indian Statistical Service) were neglected cadres. Those two cadres somewhat improved in later years. I thought myself to be lucky that I was not one of them. Thank you, *bandhwallas*, you have helped me by default.

Foreigners in the Campus

'I was not born for one corner; the whole world is my native land'
–Lucius Annaeus Seneca.

A group of seven students from various American universities came to India under the banner of World University Students Camp. They came to India for one month to know about Indian life and culture. They came to Narendrapur for more than a week. This was some time in July 1964. Bikash da selected me from our college for representing the University of Calcutta.

Watanabe, a Japanese-American, led the US team. There were three young woman students – Sue, Ellen and Babes. Besides, there was Jerry, and a very tall, six and half feet, African-American Charles. It was quite a task to find a bed for Charles. There were four students representing Jadavpur University. I was the youngest member in the group. Bada Maharaj told me to closely interact with them and help them as far as possible. This was my first exposure to American culture.

We did some fieldwork in the day like repairing a road in *Acharyaya Pally*, our Teachers' Quarters. We did some fieldwork in nearby villages as well where our Lokshiksha Parishad had a presence. One evening Ashish, a student from Jadavpur University, invited us for dinner. The family was rich and aristocratic. Their hospitality was remarkable. The lady of the house suggested that the American girls could try some Indian dresses. Sue agreed and returned after some time gorgeously dressed in a sari and gold jewelry.

This exposure helped me to mix with them more closely, learn from them about the lifestyle, education system and certain nuances of the

American culture. They also asked many questions about the diversity of Indian lifestyle and culture, the uniqueness of the vast country, poverty, so on and so forth.

Bada Maharaj dropped in sometimes. The participants' interaction with him was always very interesting. They asked him many questions about India's culture, religion, political system, economy, customs and languages. He had his charming and brief ways to answer their questions.

I became close to the group. Ellen and Jerry became good friends. They corresponded with me for quite some time. Jerry sent me some US dollar notes and coins nicely attached on a decorative piece of a cardboard for displaying in our school exhibition. They told me to come to the USA for higher studies. I dreamt about the prospect.

Some Peace Corps Volunteers came to Narendrapur to teach in the school. Peace Corps was introduced by the US President Kennedy in 1961 towards helping willing developing countries in areas of education, business, agriculture, working with non-profit organizations (NGOs) and entrepreneurs. Their duration was 24 months and several Peace Corps volunteers came to Narendrapur. The Peace Corps volunteers were 'missionaries of democracy'.

Incidentally, I read an interesting book in later years, '*The Two Year Mountain: A Nepal Journey*', written by a Peace Corps volunteer, Phil Deutschle. The book narrates the story of the young author's challenging physical and spiritual experience in a small mountain village in Nepal as a teacher. He learned Nepalese language to teach school students Science and Mathematics in their language, surviving largely on boiled rice and *dal*. He was rather critical about the implementation of the program. While in Nepal, he climbed the dangerous 20,580 feet Mount Pharchamo all by himself, risking his life. When he left after two years, the villagers were in tears.[1]

Later on several occasions, I had foreigners as my roommates. In 1966, Iain Willis, a bright student from British Colombia University, Canada, with a first class Master's in English literature became my roommate. I was in my final year MA class. I had some apprehensions about having a foreigner roommate. However, with Iain in, my apprehensions were soon gone.

Iain, a tall – over six feet – was very soft spoken albeit in a very clear voice. He arrived to render voluntary service under the Canadian Government's program equivalent to the American Peace Corps.

Even during December, Iain would take a cold water shower in the night and lie down only in his undergarment with the fan in full blast reading a collection of the Charlie Brown comic strip. He was from British Colombia, a very cold place. He felt comfortable in our winter, when the temperature would be around 12–15 degree Celsius. Reading Charlie Brown, he would sometime laugh loudly, roll over and almost fall from his bed, snapping the mosquito net. That was my first introduction to the popular Peanuts comic strip, Charlie Brown, the most 'lovable loser' created by Charles Schulz.

Iain taught English in the senior school and became very popular as he was always helping students.

We moved to the senior school hostel together as roommates. We started learning Spanish together. Iain already had an orientation in Spanish. I also had some idea about the vastness of the Spanish literature. I told Iain that I have heard: "If you are to talk business, talk in English. If you are to talk scholarship, talk in Germany. If you want to talk love, talk in Bengali or French. If you are to talk to God, speak in Spanish."

Incidentally, four of my poems were translated in Spanish and were published in a magazine from Brazil. That was possible because of my coincidental meeting with a journalist from Brazil who was a lover of India. Therefore, my interest in learning Spanish coincided with that of Iain.

Within a year's time, Iain built a good rapport with many people in Calcutta. He used to take me to the house of the director of the British Council and some other places. He came to know about the organization called Missionary Brothers of Charity, set up for the downtrodden male folks living on roads or slums. It was the male equivalent of Mother Teresa's organization. The Brothers used to live like the poor people whom they served. Iain got interested in serving them and moved out of Narendrapur.

I visited Iain in his new place. The Brothers worked in slums of Howrah, the other side of river Ganga. I had dinner with them one evening. They lived like the poor people they served – some coarse rice and dal, plus one green chili, if you liked it, as a luxury! On the weekend, he used to come to meet me at Narendrapur. I tried to take care of him. He needed a balanced and a proper diet. Eventually his health deteriorated and he had to go to Canada to his grandmother, who had raised him.

Iain returned after six months, but not to Narendrapur. He fell in love with 'Incredible' India! He gradually adopted certain Hindu rituals. He started reading about Indian culture and its heritage. He kept on visiting me frequently. We used to discuss so many things particularly about Indian culture. He loved Bengali food.

Iain was an unconventional person. He virtually gave up the conventional professional career, became involved in the social sector of India and sincerely tried to contribute his services. Our friendship deepened progressively.

Iain adopted Hindu religious practices including performing 'Yajna' – burning of chips of wood, sandal and pouring ghee into the sacred fire, simultaneously reciting the appropriate stanzas from Hindu holy scriptures, the Vedas. He came under the influence of an unconventional holy man from Pune. Subsequently, Iain left India to join Vittakivi International Center, Hauho, Finland to teach English, initially for a few months and later for a longer period. He also worked there as a gardener.

He got married to Mary, who had two kids from her first marriage, Christopher and Kim. Iain travelled to several places of India to find out what he could do. Eventually, he was involved with an NGO, working in protecting the environment. They came to stay with us in Mumbai on several occasions.

When they were in Vittakivi again, Iain and Mary received a large box of gifts for their yet to be born kid – with one hundred items of clothes and some other essential things that a new born would need, two of each item. That was a gift from the Government of Finland, welcoming the newborn! A newborn is welcome in Finland, where the birth rate is very low. Scandinavian countries like Finland, Sweden and

Norway are textbook examples of welfare states; to a certain extent, they still are!

This was the time our son was to be born. Iain returned about two months before our son's birth. Iain came with his wife and three kids – the third one was Nona. They brought exactly 50 of all those gift items that they received from the Finnish government and gave them to Tapati for our yet to be born son! Such soft, comfortable, easy to wear, and exquisitely beautiful dresses for an infant were not available in India in those days.

Iain was so much in love with India that he and Mary came to India so that their child would be born at Uttar Kashi, at the foothills of the Himalaya! He believed in reincarnation of birth. He thought that the baby would be blessed if born at a sacred place like Uttar Kashi. The baby was named Annalora.

Other foreign nationals too became my roommates. Alex Cummings came from the UK to Narendrapur School to teach English. The American Peace Corps might have inspired this British program. A perfect gentleman, Alex was my roommate in a hostel. After some months, we moved to Ramakrishnanda Bhavan where we had two separate rooms like a small flat. We used to discuss current and topical issues of our time. Alex introduced me to 'The Economist' newspaper, founded by James Wilson in 1843.

One day I saw a copy of the Ulysses by James Joyce, the Irish author. It is a story, rather the process of thoughts and actions of his main characters Leopold Bloom, Marry Bloom and other minor characters in Dublin, on a particular day, June 16 1904, written in a style called 'the stream of consciousness' in literary review. The text is … scattered and fragmented… similar to our thoughts, perceptions and memories.[2] As such, it is difficult to read and understand the book.

Alex asked me if I had read it. I told him what I remembered about it. Iain and I discussed the style of James Joyce. I admitted that I could not finish it. In fact, going through a few pages was a problem. Alex was impressed and told me, "You will have to first make up your mind to read it; if you can finish it, you will be happy."

It used to be very pleasant to sit with him to discuss current issues, an intellectually satisfying experience.

There was also Robin Martin, who was very closely involved with students.

Apart from the foreign volunteers, there was Amal da, an American, who became a monk of the Ramakrishna order. He was rector/vice principal of the school. Amal da was the quietest person I have ever seen in my life. He would speak very softly and briefly – one has to be very attentive to hear him. You could feel a sense of peace just sitting with him. He would sit in his ground floor office, attend to his academic administration works and teach English to English medium students of 10th as well as 11th standard classes. Amal da had to go back to the States for taking care of his old parents. I took him to my known tailor in Esplanade for stitching his suit. Those were the days of bell-bottom trousers with extended flares. When asked about the style of the trouser, Amal da laughed his loudest seeing a bell-bottom trouser. Obviously, he preferred conventional trousers.

Yet another American also became a monk of the Ramakrishna order. He came to Narendrapur for a very short period. He was just the opposite of Amal da. He was tall, above six feet, very smart and a great conversationalist. He lived and worked in some Latin American countries like Colombia, Brazil and Argentina. Hearing stories and anecdotes about his experiences in those countries, we used to go wild with laughter.

Then we had Hara from Japan, a very erudite and soft spoken person. He came to India to get an understanding about Indian Culture. He stayed at Narendrapur for about a year. He was regularly meeting Bada Maharaj and some other senior monks. We used to spend quite some quality time together. He was keenly interested in Indian Classical music. Soon we became friends.

When I was a child, I read a story about four Japanese kids – two boys and two girls. They came to visit a village in Bengal. I still remember the name of the team leader, O' Hara. They took a guided tour of the village where important landmarks of the village were shown to them. I kept the book with me for a long time. It opened my horizon to the country of the rising Sun. I told this story of my love for Japan to Hara and he was very happy.

Pandit Ravi Shankar, the Sitar maestro, sometimes used to come to Narendrapur. He was very close to our Kalipada da. One evening, we saw them talking on the road in front of Bramhanannda Bhavan. Next day there was an announcement in the press that Panditji would be performing at Ravindra Sadan. Hara wanted to go and we booked minimum priced tickets. We had to sit on the crowded first floor balcony, where from we could neither see Panditji properly nor hear him playing.

I thought of a plan and told Hara about it. Hara occasionally contributed to *Ashahi Simbun*. I saw his visiting card. The card was written in Japanese. Hara also had an impressive looking Yashica camera. I told him that we could take a chance. We went near the stage from the rear entrance and someone stopped us. I told the person, "My friend Hara is from Japan. He occasionally contributes to a leading daily in Tokyo. If we can stand somewhere near the stage, we will be very obliged." He asked me, "And who are you?" I told him that I was from the Ramakrishna Mission, Narendrapur. By then three, four others had gathered and were listening to our conversation. An important sounding person looked at the card with a confused expression. I explained and Hara as always stood with folded palms in a perpetual bowing position, occasionally adjusting the sling of the camera so that it was noticed. The man helped us to go near the dais.

After the performance was over, Hara took a number of photographs of Panditji and his associates and instruments. He gave us autographs. When we went out and walked some distance, Hara tried to look for words to express his gratitude. Eventually he managed to tell me in broken English, "I was in heaven for the last four hours! It is all because of you. I got this wonderful time of my life. I shall definitely publish some of the photographs and a short report about Panditji's performance." He repeatedly thanked me. We reached Narendrapur when dawn was about to break.

I shall close this chapter with Jim and Bacha. They came by car all the way from Sweden. As a couple, they looked somewhat odd. Jim was much older to Bacha. The name Bacha was derived from Bengali

Baccha, meaning a kid. Bacha's father was Swedish and mother Bengali. Bacha's mother was living all by herself in Calcutta. As a person, she was a committed Gandhian, even in her style of living.

Jim was a painter and Bacha was a student of medicine. They came to India driving straight from Stockholm to Calcutta. That was a fantastic journey, filled with joy, laughter, scare and danger. They were guests at Indian Statistical Institute, Calcutta when Tapati and I were doing a course in the mid June 1971. We became friends.

After a few days, they moved to St Paul's Cathedral, where foreign tourists used to get camping facility for a few days. Hearing their adventurous story about their long journey, Bada Maharaj invited Jim to stay a few days in Narendrapur. Bacha was staying with her mother. One day Jim and I went to meet Bacha's mother. The lady was living in her own small house, but her living room was very spacious. It was filled with so many things – artifacts, paintings, ceramic objects, and what not. Within a short time, she held me close to her, as if we knew each other for long! She touched my head and blessed me like a mother.

When I moved to Mumbai, they came, stayed with me for a week. My old aunt was staying with me at that time. They became friends with my old aunt. My aunt was a great host and highly hospitable. I heard from her that in our house in Hasail, no visitor could leave without a meal. It just happened that when they were with us, I had to go to Pune to take part in a management course for three days at Tata Management Training Centre (TMTC). I could go because they assured me of taking care of my aunt. My aunt also agreed without any hesitation. Our young housekeeper from Calcutta assured me to do her best.

On my return, I heard from all four of them that they had a great time together. I still have a photograph with beaming faces of all of them. If the heart was willing, language was no barrier for communication at all!

The Difficult Sixties

The flight has been moving towards Iceland; within a few hours, it will enter the Scandinavian sky. My mouth is dry. I am thirsty. Is it dehydration? I know that travel by air can shed up to 1.5 litres of water from body during an average three-hour flight!

I moved over to senior section school, i.e., from ninth to 11th standards in 1968 as full time teacher of Economics and Social Studies as well as house master in the hostel. I was moving with the same batch of students from sixth to 11th standard. My salary was Rs. 560 consolidated. Besides, as a house master my boarding and lodging was on the school account. This, however, was not a 'job' per say. I was passionately involved in various activities of the ashram.

The business environment in West Bengal was getting from bad to worse. There were *gheraos, bandhs, dharmaghats* and strikes. Almost every day there were processions on the streets of Calcutta. By 1968, the CPI (ML) led Naxalite movement was gaining ground. Killing people became easy as well as remorseless and cops started hounding young people.

Despite his illness, my father told me not to leave Narendrapur unless I got a job to my satisfaction in terms of compensation, safety and convenience of location. I made more frequent visits to see my father and aunt. Just after one visit in early July, 1969, I came back to Narendrapur. It was difficult to take leave from school when classes were going on. The next day, our neighbor's son came with news that my father was not feeling well at all. I had to rush. Something from inside told me that I was going to bid him farewell. On my way home from the station, I dropped in at the doctor's house. He told me that my father was in his last stages and it was good that I had come. I sat by him for a few hours. His suffering was acute and I held his hand tight and stroked his hairs, they still were black. So many memories of him came rushing to my mind like flash back scenes in a movie.

In the midnight, my father breathed his last after a couple of coughing bouts. I could not believe my eyes. Seeing him dead, I remembered my mother's death. At that time, I was a kid. I did not understand that she was dead. I saw and heard with great puzzle that everybody present suddenly started crying and howling. In front of my own eyes, I saw my father's living body become absolutely still, no movement at all! Gradually, his body became cold. Just in a few seconds, my father became his body! Death! Death came stealthily on to him.

The indomitable fighting man, my loving father, had at last decided to go to bed. Now I would have to take care of my old aunt. In the absence of my mother, she took care of my sister, father and me. We would have been lost without her.

I faced so many odd things in one small life that I became somewhat hardened. Yet tears came like the flow of a fountain from nowhere. For several hours, I was without voice, without words. I just shed tears and tears. My last biological link with nature, or should I say universe, was snapped. I was now alone in this world.

Suppressing my emotion, I had to get up and arrange for the cremation. Neighbors were all there to help. We took him to the naturally made crematorium, about a kilometer away, under a large bushy tree. I lit the pyre, the second time in my life, but this time on my father's face.

Take rest, at last take some rest in peace, my dear father! You fought so gallantly. Success went away like a mirage from you. Despite deteriorating health, you continued your fight round after round after the partition for saving us from poverty, illness and for giving us a comfortable living as far as possible.

At last, when nothing worked, you took the right decision to bring us to Dhubilia. You ensured our survival without losing dignity. Since the partition made us refugees for no fault of ours, living for a certain period on Government doles as a last resort was understandable. With dignity and clear mind, he told me, and I wholeheartedly agreed with him, that we must not go in for the so-called rehabilitation program of the Government again. He left the baton for me to take up, and run and win the race.

The ritual of organizing the *Shraddha* ceremony was performed. My aunt Santi, uncle Bhabaranjan's wife, and cousin Sankar came from Calcutta to Dhubulia for a couple of days to attend the last rites as well as offer their love and respect to my father. It was really an attribute, an expression of genuine love and affection for my father. They were well off people. Usually people belonging to higher strata in society would not like to stay in Dhubulia even for a day. They were different, they were humans with good feelings and good souls. They came for my father who must have been something important and dear to them. I felt happy and relaxed. I was not alone in the world after all.

I went back to Narendrapur after a few days. The routine work in the school and hostel had to be carried on. I promised my aunt to drop in once in a fortnight.

On a request from National Council of Educational Research and Training (NCERT) to Bada Maharaj, I had to go to Delhi to take part in a workshop for restructuring the curriculum of Social Studies at the all India level. That was my first ever trip to Delhi. During my studies at the Masters level, I had been too many places in India as part of our education tour. This was different in the sense that Bada Maharaj considered me fit to go to a workshop organized by NCERT for revising the content of Social Studies at higher secondary level. There was one Dr. Mehta who was the organizer. I am sorry that I have forgotten his first name. He was fair complexioned, of medium height and a smart person. He took me into confidence as the youngest member, sent by Swami Lokeswarananda to whom he was very respectful.

After the first round of deliberation, I got the responsibility of drafting the first cut of the revised curriculum of Social Studies. I spent many hours in the night to write and rewrite several versions. Eventually, by early morning my draft came up to my satisfaction. In the next meeting, members discussed and revised the draft prepared by me. They complemented me and Dr. Mehta congratulated me. The revised curriculum later became a document of NCERT.

I was happy. My father would have been happier to know that I had successfully performed my delegated responsibility.

Dr. Mehta had a passion for national integration. He suggested that we should organize a students' camp in Narendrapur with mixed groups of students coming from various states of India. He wrote to Bada Maharaj about it.

With the help of Parameswer da and some other teachers, I organized the students' national integration camp for three days during Diwali vacation in the junior school campus in 1969. Students and teachers from Punjab, Tamil Nadu and Maharashtra participated. I invited Dr. Mehta, but he could not make it. With funding from NCERT, the camp was very successful. Many students and teachers, who came from various states kept in touch with me, writing letters and inviting me to their places. Dr. Mehta was very happy about the success of the camp.

Time moved on. A protest by manual laborers like cooks, helpers, people working in the poultry and dairy firms was organized by CPI (M) in June 1970 in our institute. The strike continued for over a month. A workers' union was hastily formed. They wanted a pay hike and recognition of their newly formed union with outside leadership.

We had to cook breakfast, lunch and dinner for about 1,500 students and teachers as well as other residents staying in the campus every day in eight kitchens attached to school and college hostels. Groceries and other materials used to be supplied at night. To milk the cows, a dozen dairy workers were quietly sent by P.C. Sen, former Chief Minister. The striking workers together with their recently found leaders raised slogans every day near the main gate.

In our internal meetings, I had been taking a sympathetic stance for considering a certain pay hike in the presence of the leaders of the newly formed union. At the same time, I did not agree with their demand for very a huge raise and recognition of their union with outside political leadership. There was a court verdict that educational institutes could not have 'trade unions' with outside political leadership as in a company.

It was difficult to go out of the campus. Classes in the school and college were held in an irregular manner. Cooking food became the main activity. There were occasional meetings with the leaders of the union and the ashram team. I took part in these meetings on behalf of the ashram.

The demand was to raise the pay scale to an abnormally high level. Prior to this, such a strike was organized in Sibpur Engineering College, now a university. The same was in IIT, Khargpur. The union leaders also demanded 'trade union' status for workers' union in educational institutions. From our side, certain reasonable pay hike was offered. The local MLA, belonging to CPI (M) was the leader. He refused to accept any offer and insisted on fulfillment of all their demands and formal recognition of the newly formed workers' union.

After discussing with Bada Maharaj, Pransankar da (Dr. Pran Shankar Chakraborty, Professor of Geology, Jadavpur University) and I went to meet Comrade Jyoti Basu, former Deputy Chief Minister at his residence, Hindustan Park Road, Gariahata, South Calcutta. He led a spartan life as we could see from the sitting room. There was a modest sofa, a small table and a few chairs in the small living room. He received us courteously. We appraised him about the strike.

Mr. Basu heard both of us. He promised to intervene. In any case, he was respectful to Bada Maharaj and sympathetic to the activities of Ramakrishna Mission, Narendrapur, even though he was a staunch Communist.

Within a few days, the workers came back on their own to resume their work. The strike fizzled out. Some of us had been requesting the management for implementing the raise in pay scale and not to victimize leaders of the agitation. The management of the institute gave them a pay raise, but there was some victimization also. We got to know about that later.

In those days, there was Army and police posting in the campus. Combing operations were going on to trace out Naxalite youth, guns and handmade bombs. Many young persons were arrested. Tons of literature had been written on the Naxalite movement of Bengal… I am not repeating them here.

The base office of the temporary Army camp was in our gymnasium building. It was under the command of one Major. They used to help local cops in combing operations. The Major used to attend the institute's cultural functions. We became very friendly. Within a couple of weeks, normalcy was restored. Our campus became peaceful again

The decade of the 1960s was a difficult time for the society in general and Indian economy in particular as I have already mentioned. Many foreign experts ruled out the 'concept' of India. During that time, we experienced job scarcity too.

Quite unexpectedly, China attacked India in October 1962 and virtually took over what was then known as North Eastern Frontier Area, rechristened as Arunachal later. Apprehension was that perhaps Assam would fall into Chinese hands. Pandit Nehru was shocked and depressed. He took it as a betrayal by a friendly neighbor. His health deteriorated. His efforts towards building friendly relationship with China fell apart, although initially China also warmly responded to his overtures. The '*Hindi – Chini Bhai Bhai*' song and dance lost its sheen.

The McMahon Line, based on a treaty between Britain and Tibet in 1914, demarcated the border between India and China. However, the McMahon Line was not acceptable to the Peoples' Republic of China. China 'aggressed' Tibet in 1950–51. During the Tibetan Uprising in 1959, His Holiness the 14th Dalai Lama left Tibet, fearing that his life was in danger, and reached India. Eventually, about 80,000 Tibetan refugees came to India. They have been living as 'refugees' at Dharamasla, Himachal Pradesh, where Dalai Lama has formed his Government of Tibet in Exile.

The effect of the Chinese aggression also hit the Indian economy adversely. As the Indian military's war preparedness was found to be wanting, several measures were taken. NCC was made compulsory. In spite of my taking Military Studies at the Inter level where NCC was my 'practical' paper, I had to be enrolled again in NCC in my first year BA honors course. But, the kind of facilities, including full set of uniforms that we received earlier was not available after NCC was made compulsory due to shortage of funds.

There was yet another war. During April to September 1965, border skirmishes were going on with West Pakistan. Then, in response to Pakistan's "Operation Gibraltar' – to infiltrate Jammu and Kashmir and start a war against India – a full-fledged Indo-Pak war started in August 1965.

Sandbags were placed in our main buildings in Narendrapur. In the evening windows were pasted with newspapers so that the ray of light was not visible to the outside world. NCC parades were going on with great vigor. People were collecting donations, both in cash and kind, including jewelry to be sent to appropriate authorities. The patriotic feeling was loud and clear.

The effect of this war was felt seriously on the economy. There was a severe drought in 1965–66. There was massive food shortage. The USA announced the PL 480 aid and wheat started arriving from the USA. Rice particularly was in short supply, so *chapatis or fulkas* were served at lunch and dinner.

In those days, Bengalis did not like *chapatis* at all. I remember that in our hostels when *chapatis* were served for the first time, there were tears in the eyes of students. To make *chapatis* attractive, mutton was served with them. Some of us teachers in school as well as house masters in the hostels took only *chapatis* and no rice meals to set an example. To be honest, we also did not like it then. When I look back now, I feel how stupid we were all. Over a period, *chapatis* have become an essential item in the daily Bengali menu.

Lal Bahadur Shastri, a simple and straightforward Gandhian, who believed in Nehruvian socialism and non-alignment, was our second Prime Minister after the death of Jawaharlal Nehru on May 27, 1964. He introduced the '*Jai Jawan, Jai Kishan*' slogan. He requested people to fast one day in the week to save food. Many people heeded his request and did fast one day in a week.

The war ended in January when the Tashkent Agreement was signed between India and Pakistan on January 10, 1966. Lal Bahadur Shastri was at Tashkent to sign the treaty. He died of a heart attack on the following night at Tashkent.

During this difficult period of 1965 and 1966, we were in our Masters classes. Those were the days of food shortage. The food situation in West Bengal in those days was very difficult. Chief Minister P.C. Sen advised people to include green banana of a particular species to their diet, as it was nutritious. He was ridiculed. He also banned sweet products within the municipal limits of Calcutta. That was due to shortage of milk. Bengalis love sweets. There were large varieties of sweets made and consumed in Bengal. Many exquisite sweets are made today, which have become a lifestyle statement of Bengalis. The honest, albeit austere, move of P.C. Sen was negated by a mushroom growth of sweet shops just outside the city limit.

Food production in India declined by an average 2.2% during the first half of 1960s. The growth somewhat moved up to 2.5% during the second half. Food grains production was just 82 million tons during 1960–61 and moved up to 108.4 million tons in 1970–71. The figure increased to 264.8 million tons in 2013–14. At the same time, the rate of consumer price (industrial workers) inflation was slowly increasing, 0.9% during the mid-1950s to around 6.5% during the 1960s. Overall the national income growth during the 1960s was less than 3%; with per capita income at a less than 1%.[1] It was catastrophe all around.

There was acute shortage of foreign exchange. The current account deficits were paid initially by drawing on the Pound Sterling balance left by the British India government. This was a negative example of consuming and depleting your 'capital', instead of using it to create assets. The overvalued rupee was to be devalued by 57% from the Rs. 4.76 to Rs. 7.50 per US $ on July 6, 1966.

The end of the decade saw vigorous socialist initiatives by Indira Gandhi, which continued in the early 1970s after the Bangladesh War of Independence. Indira Gandhi played a courageous role by deploying Indian forces for directly helping the war efforts of the Mukti Sena of Bangladesh.

At the same time, she introduced a robust socialist orientation in her economic and business policies. She appointed a number of Left politicians and ideologues to advise her, including, for example our teacher Dr. Ashok Mitra. The managing agency system was abolished, banks were nationalized, restrictions of monopoly were introduced, and the group concept of large houses was withdrawn.

The disturbing decade of the 1960s transcended into an extraordinary situation when India got directly involved, and rightly so, in helping the

Independence War of Bangladesh in 1971 as discussed elsewhere. Prime Minister Indira Gandhi travelled all over the world seeking help from powerful countries but returned empty handed. Soviet Russia as usual stood by, while President Nixon, not a friend of India, sent the Seventh Fleet to the Bay of Bengal to create pressure on India. Fortunately, good sense prevailed and the fleet was withdrawn. Indira Gandhi's courage stood out among the league table of the world's political leaders. India helped Bangladesh to become Independent. Moreover, India had to receive and take care of 10 million refugees.

CHAPTER 16

Moving to Outside World

Thoughts and images of my early days have been moving fast on my mental screen. Somehow, I am in a daze. The pilot is addressing… the plane is flying above 35,000 feet altitude and temperature outside is minus 54 degree Celsius. I tried to comprehend how cold that would be – no way; but in Russia's Yakutia region, the temperature could drop to minus 67 degree Celsius. People also live there!

More than two decades had passed after we moved from East Bengal. We have moved from one place to the other so frequently that I lost count. Coming to Narendrapur gave me a long breathing space. I already completed more than a decade there. I had not stayed anywhere else for such a long time. I consider myself lucky, despite so many hassles that I faced.

Some of my batch mates hailed from East Bengal and came straight to the refugee camp and then to Narendrapur. They did not have to move so frequently like me. They got settled one way or the other. That was certainly a step forward from the days of partition. The next generation, my generation, took over the mantle.

Some of those who could not enter Narendrapur also completed their schooling in the camp, and subsequently moved out of the camps by opting for rehabilitation. Initially they did some sundry jobs or started small businesses like starting a retail shop or trading. A smaller number of them also continued their education in evening colleges. Girls also took advantage of school education in a big way. The bright ones went further and completed their graduation. Some of them entered nursing courses and became nurses. The graduated ones took up teaching in schools or some other small jobs. They stared earning and helping their families. More determined ones, both boys and girls, went for postgraduate education, suffering many odds – shoddy clothes, inadequate food, no electricity in the house or books, yet they pursued clenching their teeth. Many succeed in their endeavors.

Sometimes, the eldest son or daughter became the source of earning for the family. The harsh reality was that their families, parents and siblings exploited them particularly.

It is also true that if partition did not take place so many students, both boys, and more so girls, might not have developed the motivation to educate themselves. This, however, is no justification for the partition.

Their lives in refuge colonies moved on towards somewhat better and certainly more dignified ways of living than staying in the camp and living on doles. Effects of partition had a continuing impact on all our lives.

Despite his failing health, my father, after partition, wanted to live with dignity and tried out several options. Those options did not materialize, and I certainly do not blame him for that. I have my complete love and respect for him, even though we had to move from one odd place to another, despite his attempts for trying out one or the other option. And he is no more.

During the period of four years after my Masters, I was engaged in teaching in the senior section of the school. As advised by the Principal of our college, Bikash da, I took a batch of about 35 college students to work in a camp in a rural area. It was a village, Boral, just 3 kms from Garia, but not connected by tar road. During monsoon, the road turned mucky. I heard that Satyajit Ray shot certain scenes of his famous 'Panther Panchali' in that village. We built a road of about half a km in two weeks' time. Our menu was more or less like that of the local people, who were poor, except a few families. We dressed very ordinarily so that we could be close to them. We mingled with villagers very closely and tried to understand their problems. Alongside the road, we constructed a few toilets from burnt earthen rings. Those were for demonstration purposes. That was required for the people as even relatively well-off families used to relieve themselves in the open. We went from door to door to explain to them the need for the use of toilets. That was almost half a century before Prime Minister Narendra Modi initiated his nationwide campaign, *Swachha Bharat,* and popularizing use of toilets is one aspect of this program.

All families of the village invited us for lunch one day, one of us in each family. There was a rich Muslim family. They wanted to invite me for lunch. The young son of the family had joined us in the program. He became very close to me and the relationship sustained for a long time. I explained that the preference should go to students, as food offered by them would be great. I went to the poorest family in the village. I shall never forget that lunch. When I reached their hut, the man of the house climbed the coconut tree like a smart monkey, cut a few green coconuts, and came down. He sliced a few green coconuts and offered me the smooth and slightly sweet tender coconut water as well as the soft and thick pulp from around the inner walls of the shell, which was delicious. Along with it, I was served some puffed rice and chunk of clean *Gur* (jaggery). The husband, wife and kids were very happy that the camp commander had visited their house. I offered them a box of sweets, a Bengali custom when you visit a family. A divine smile spread across their faces and the children enjoyed the sweet. I still remember their smiling faces.

I also took one batch of our school students to a rural camp somewhere near Gobardanga, if I remember the name of the place correctly. Our Lokshiksha Parishad's activities were conducted by Nandadulal da, who got closely involved with the Parishad activities right from the beginning when Barun da initiated the program. There also we built a road, which would last long. Many visitors including the press visited the camp and reported our work in newspapers. Some foreign guests also came along with Bada Maharaj. We used to organize cultural functions every evening. The villagers were very happy and mingled with us as if we all belonged to a large family. Two incidents happened, one before the camp and the other during the camp.

One was unique. In my hostel, there was Nikhil (not real name), a very intelligent student, but naughty. He was very strong in language and literature and could write brilliantly for his age. His mischievous activities irritated some teachers and students. He would speak sweetly with a measured tune and logical flow. He could lie smoothly without batting an eyelid. He would always appear convincing. He would create trouble for those teachers who would scold or punish him. He would not also spare fellow students who complained against him for his misdeeds.

On a couple of occasions when I interrogated Nikhil, Barun da, then headmaster of the school, sat there, counting Nikhil's pulse movements. Barun da told me later that he was checking pulse beats and studying his face to understand whether Nikhil was lying or not.

His official guardian was one of his parents. Apparently, the family was estranged, parents separated. Sometimes the other parent came to visit alone to meet Nikhil. With Nikhil in the class or in the hostel, there never could be a dull moment. He would do one mischief or another.

If something out of the way happened in the hostel, I could feel the vibration that something was wrong. I used to quietly watch, follow movements and stray words of boys. One afternoon I felt something big was going on. I heard someone saying, "let's go to the study hall." That was not the time to go to the study hall, which was on the third floor.

I rushed quietly to the next hostel building where from the study hall of our hostel was visible. I noticed that eight/ 10 students had encircled someone, and some angry noise was heard. I went straight to the study hall of our hostel on the third floor. They certainly did not expect me to be there. "Oh! Jiban da! How do you always turn up when we do not expect you," the students asked

"What's going on," I asked. One leader answered, "We were coming to you with Nikhil." I heard the story, which appeared absurd. I spoke to Nikhil alone, "I heard everything, Nikhil, and I think what they said is right. Do you realize that you are involved in serious misconduct?"

Nikhil's head was hung low. Quietly he went to my desk, took a sheet of paper and wrote down his confession. I do not want to reveal what the misconduct was; that is not important here.

I was shocked and surprised beyond my wits by reading his confession. I had to discuss this with the headmaster. This made us to call Nikhil's mother. Sudhanshu Maharaj, an erudite monk, was headmaster of the senior school for a short period. When we were talking to the boy's mother in the headmaster's office, the father also walked in quite unexpectedly. When he saw his estranged wife, he was about to rush out. Sudhanshu da got up from his seat and called him in. It was an embarrassing situation for both of them. Sudhanshu da gave a precise and impact-making emotional talk to both the parents. I also spoke. Eventually, we told them to consider coming together for the interest of their teenage son. They tentatively agreed. The boy was in tears and we consoled him.

It was an issue whether we should take him to the social work camp or not. The camp was scheduled to be held after two days. I was uncomfortable to leave Nikhil alone in the hostel. Despite all his wrong doings, I admired his creative side. We often spoke about so many things. He was a great company. He could write well and paint well. I sincerely wanted him to be a great success in life. He had all the potential to be a successful person. At the same time, he had great talent for mischief making. I spoke to him frankly and took a pledge that he would behave in the camp.

One afternoon in the camp, we saw, with our eyes bobbling out, that Nikhil's parents came together with a huge basket of sweet. There was a celebration all around. The powerful counseling by Sudhanshu da made all this to happen.

I remember him telling me, "Jiban, I am a monk first, then a headmaster. Let us make an attempt if we can help the parents to build a bridge." The attempt was successful. I wished Shudhansu da were there to witness the success of his intervention. It was my great pleasure to meet and interact with him when he was head of the library in Ramakrishna math in Santacruz, Mumbai in later years.

The other incident was in fact an accident averted. In the village, there was a large pond on which dried water hyacinth made a thick carpet above the water. If you were lightweight, you could run fast on the padded carpet and get to the other shore. However, if you stood still even for a few seconds you would gradually sink. Then it would be beyond retrieval.

The area was made out of bounds for students in the camp. Nevertheless, one student made a quiet visit there after lunch. He started running, got scared and stood there bewildered and was about to go down. Some elderly villagers saw that and raised a clamor. They hesitated in deciding what to do. Some people called us. I rushed to the scary scene. My NCC training was of help. Seeing me running some young village boys also joined me. Without thinking anything, we ran fast, held the boy's hand and told him to run fast with us. For a moment, he was not sure. The village boys were shouting instructions. We all ran fast to the nearest shore. We made it. The boy was about to faint. We all were in a state of trance. After sometime there was huge merriment. Almost all campers were there to celebrate. I still feel scared thinking of the incident. It could have been a disaster.

On the day of our return, the village women stood in two lines throwing flower petals as we moved on. Some blew conch shells and tears flowed down their cheeks. Our eyes were also misty and we waved on as long they were in our sight. It was a wonderful experience. People in the Bengal villages do have golden hearts. If only the developmental paradigm had transformed their socio-economic plight, the situation would have been different on a rich ground with immense potential.

Dr. Radha Kamal Mukherjee, an eminent economist, passed out from the very first batch of students getting Masters' degree in Economics from Calcutta University. His brother, Radha Kumud, was an eminent historian. Dr. Radha Kamal Mukherjee came to Narendrapur for almost a month during summer vacation as Bada Maharaj's guest. Bada Maharaj requested me to help him with his academic project. Dr. Mukherjee was preparing a draft proposal for a World University to be set up by the United Nations. From breakfast to lunch he would work, largely giving me dictation and occasionally breaking into talking. After lunch, he would take an hour's rest and read my handwritten scripts and from 3 p.m. to 5 p.m., he would again give dictation. That was the routine for every day.

He was fair complexioned, medium height and thin. He used to wear a light ghee colored full-sleeved shirt on a more or less same colored trouser with a Gandhi cap on his head. He spoke in an elegant voice; his words would flow like a smooth waterfall, precise and logical. He became a role model for me.

He asked me many questions about my family, my background and all that. It was privilege to have received his love and affection.

He was then Director, J.K. Institute of Research, Lucknow University. Before leaving the campus, he told me that I should do PhD on slum re-development related issues under him in Lucknow. I still remember him saying, "Slum brutalizes humanity..." He gave me a number of reading material and asked me to go to Lucknow after three months. I kept in touch with him. However, as my bad luck would have it, he suddenly expired! My first chance for doing PhD died with him.

I had applied to participate in a three-week course on Research Methodology, organized under the sponsorship of Indian Council for Research in Social Science (ICSSR) to be held at Indian Statistical Institute (ISI), Calcutta during summer vacation in 1971. I was accepted to attend the course as I was already enrolled to do PhD under S.B. Mukherjee, Chief Economist, Calcutta Metropolitan Planning Organization (CMPO). Dr. S.N. Sen, then Vice Chancellor, Calcutta University, suggested me to go to S.B. Mukherjee, who was an expert on demography and related areas, and worked on census data. He was a nice, sweet speaking person, tall and slim with a deep voice. He heard my experience with Dr. Radha Kamal Mukherjee and eventually accepted me after a couple of rounds of talks and advised me to read some books and reports. I used to go to the CMPO library. In those days, Ford Foundation mentored CMPO. The Basic Development of Calcutta Plan was prepared by the CMPO in the late 1960s at the instance of Dr. B.C. Roy, Chief Minister.

About 20 participants attended the course. Among the faculty members, there were big names like Prof. Moni Mukherjee, one of the pioneers of India's nation income accounts, Dr. Nikhilesh Bhattacharyay, Dr. D.K. Basu, Dr. Ashok Rudra and several others. It was a residential program. We stayed at the ESIC hostel. This was the only time in my life that I got an opportunity to concentrate on learning. For me the course was extremely useful, particularly to learn quantitative methods for conducting research projects.

I also had the opportunity to interact with several faculty members. I was very much interested to know more about national accounts in general and that of India in particular. I sought appointment with Prof.

Moni Mukherjee and attended some sessions. I got to know him better later in my life.

A visiting professor at our graduation level initiated my interest in the subject. A young Dr. Banerjee took some sessions on national income accounts though that was not on our syllabus of the Honors course. Later in my life when I was an economist with the Tata Group, I had the opportunity to follow up the subject when I became a member, and later an executive Committee member of the Indian Association of Research in National Income and Wealth (IARNIW).

Above all, it was there I first met Tapati, a vibrant and spontaneously smart person, my future partner of life.

Coming back to Narendrapur, I realized that I would have to follow up further education in the field of research methodology. Opportunity came from the Council for Social Development (CSD), New Delhi where an advance course on the subject would be organized in October 1971 with ICSSR sponsorship. Since I took the first such course in ISI Calcutta, I was accepted for the advanced course. It was a course for over two weeks organized by CSD, located next to the beautiful campus of India International Center (IIC), the venue of Delhi's top intellectuals, socialites, VIPs of all shapes and shades. We stayed at the IIPS hostel at Indraprasta area in New Delhi. The spectacular office of Ford Foundation was also in the campus of the famous India International Center. The World Bank India office was on the first floor of CSD. It was a magnificent cluster of reputed institutions in one eye catching beautiful campus. I had the opportunity to explore resources from all those establishments. For me, it was another worldly experience.

Dr. C. D. Deshmukh, a former ICS officer, established the IIC. He was the first Indian Governor of Reserve Bank of India in 1943. Dr. Deshmukh was also Finance Minister in Nehru's cabinet during 1950–56. He built several institutions like IIC. Despite all such glorifying past, Dr. Deshmukh was a very humble person. Never ever, did he show any pompous attitude. His second wife Durgabai Deshmukh, an eminent freedom fighter, social worker, lawyer, was a member of the Constituent Assembly of India as well as the Planning Commission of India and was a formidable lady.

She was the spirit behind establishing the CSD. Dr. Pradipta Roy, a reputed Social Scientist, was the then Director of CSD. Several competent faculty members were there in CSD. A number of eminent resource persons were also invited. There was Dr. Jerry Hursh, Director of UNICEF, one of our core faculty members, who eventually became my mentor.

In the inaugural session, Dr. Deshmukh and Mrs. Deshmukh were also present along with Dr. Roy and other faculty members and some eminent experts in the field of social science research. We introduced ourselves. When I told that I had come from Ramakrishna Mission, Narendrapur, Mrs. Deshmukh promptly asked me, "How is Swami Lokeswarananda?" After I answered, she asked me some more questions about Ramakrishna Mission, Narendrapur. At the end, she told me to see her after the session.

We did both theoretical lessons as well as practical fieldwork such as hands on sample surveys in a nearby village of Haryana. We learnt how to prepare a structured questionnaire and how to establish rapport with respondents. We did the survey and prepared a report. At every stage, there was useful guidance provided by competent resource persons.

On the social side, there was an invitation for Dr. Roy's wedding dinner. We came to know that Mrs. Deshmukh had herself cooked some of the items. That was my first classy dinner where sumptuous South Indian delicacies were served.

Then there was a party thrown by Dr. Jerry Harsh on a weekend at his residence. Dr. Harsh was a very erudite person and an excellent teacher. He encouraged us to ask questions or make comments. Usually, many of my co-participants were shy. In fact, I experienced it also later that Indians suffer from a mental block of opening up in formal sessions. Despite coxing, many people would hardly speak. In any case, I made use of the opportunity. As a result, he used to call me after each session and we talked a lot. Obviously, he asked me about my background and my aspirations. For the first time, I saw a scientific calculator, which he was using. My first experience of taking a photocopy was also in his office in Ford Foundation.

When he asked me specifically about my plan, I told him that I had applied to some American Universities for MS admission. He wrote a letter of recommendation to his friend, who was a professor in a reputed American University. He read out the recommendation part of the letter, indicating my strengths and couple of weaknesses. I was grateful. Subsequently, I received admission offer with a partial scholarship. I could not go due to certain compelling circumstances.

I wrote to him about it and he understood. I sent him my marriage invitation. The letter he wrote in response was with so much warmth that my eyes filled with tears. I understood sometimes in life you come across such a good friend, who tries to smoothen the passage of your journey.

The second advanced course, also organized by CSD in 1972 with ICSSR sponsorship, was on the training on the first generation of computers. We received training on punch card system and related issues. Some of us developed quite some expertise in the punch card process. Besides, we did a survey based research project on food adulteration in certain areas of New Delhi.

Both those courses on quantitative techniques in social science research methodology including conducting a sample survey and report writing equipped us with a skill set that was not in our university curriculum. Such courses were not there in our Economics masters curriculum. Therefore, those two courses were extremely useful to me. They helped me to gain an edge in quantitative methods. I also made many friends across India and established close personal relationships with many eminent persons. Those courses gave me a drive to move ahead.

CHAPTER 17

Expanding the Horizon

The Air India's Jumbo jet Boeing 747 is flying at 575 miles (925 kms) mph. The Concord, the retired supersonic transport, had a maximum cruising speed of 1,354 miles (2,179 kms) mph. The Concord could have covered the distance between JFK and Mumbai in just six hours compared to 16 hours by Boeing. The round trip fare from New York to London by the Concord was $7,995 in 1997, 30 times the cheapest option.

During my last two years of stay in Narendrapur (1971 and 1972), I was fully involved in outside activities and realized my strength, weakness and confidence in certain areas.

To my surprise, I received an invitation in the summer vacation of 1972 from Leslie Sawhney Program for Training in Democracy (LSPTD), Mumbai to participate in a two-week course to be held at the National Institute of Training in Industrial Engineering (NITIE) campus, Andheri East, Mumbai. My surprise was because I had not heard of the organization and I also did not apply. Most exciting was the fact I would not have to pay for expenses except travel. Probably some influential person – one of my well-wishers – must have recommended me.

I reached Mumbai by train. We stayed in the new hostel of NITIE. The course started the next morning with physical exercise conducted by Lt Col Chandravadkar (Retd). Since my first romance was Army, I was able to establish a rapport with the Lt Col. Sessions began with an introduction by Arvind Deshpande, secretary, LSPTD. I came to know that LSPTD was a NGO, established in the memory of Lt Col Sawhney. He was married to J.R.D. Tata's sister. Then spoke Minoo Masani, a multi-dimensional and flamboyant personality. I was vaguely aware of his various roles from being one of the Founding Fathers of the Constitution of India to being a lawyer, corporate executive, diplomat, politician, journalist and educator. To my understanding, his political ideology was what we loosely call 'rightist'. In fact, he was a member of the Communist Party of India for a short period, moved to be socialist and eventually went to the other side of the pole. After his talk on the spirit of democracy, the Swatantraite right-oriented economic philosophy, there was a question and answer session. I asked the first question, followed by several complementary questions. He answered them and told me to see him after the session. I talked to him later at length and he advised me to read a number of books. One book he recommended was, 'The Road to Serfdom' by Friedrich Hayek. His focused and clear-cut views were of course rightist, but I wondered why Nobel laureate Hayek had to spend so much of his precious time in criticizing Lord Keynes, the most significant economist of the 20th century.

Reading various schools of thought is helpful to develop an objective perspective of one's own. Later in my life, I developed my understanding in Economics in a clear-cut manner. As a student of Economics, I have been influenced by New Keynesian theory – which evolved from Keynesianism to Neo Keynesianism, and then to New Keynesianism. I believe that there has to be a combination of supply and demand forces as well as a strong and positive role of the Government. The Government must intervene in the case of market failure by responding appropriately to move the economy up; and then it should retreat once the recovery is restored.

At the same time, I strongly believe that in a vast and largely poor country like India, the Government has a direct role to play in the economy for attaining a number of socio-economic objectives like poverty eradication, improvement of basic amenities like housing, education and health as well as engaging in utilities sectors like road, transport and energy.

There are many examples of Government intervention in case of market failure even in the so-called capitalist countries. During the Great Depression of the 1930s, President Franklin D. Roosevelt introduced with the Keynesian New Deal measures like public investment to create employment and income. It helped the American economy to move up. Even at the time of The Great Recession of the mid 2008, President Barack Obama did a massive Government intervention to restore the health of the economy.

The Chinese model of 'socialist market economy' works in case of Communist China. In case of India, we have to develop our own model. This point needs a separate discussion.

Nevertheless, I was happy to have interacted with Minoo Masani. Later, I developed a close personal relationship over years, despite differences of opinions and views. Some of his views were too idiosyncratic and not always realistic. Some economists used to say that 'some' low rate of inflation should be good for developing countries. Masani sharply criticized such observations saying in his idiosyncratic style, "...some inflation is like some pregnancy!"

Yet another sharp and outspoken resource person was Brigadier John Dalvi (Retd), who spoke after lunch on various issues relating to international relations. Tall and strongly built, Brig Dalvi spoke in a no nonsense style. He wrote the well-known book '*The Himalayan Blunder*'.

The book, initially banned in India, was an 'angry truth about India's most crushing disaster'. It is the sad story of India's inadequate military preparedness as exposed at the time of the Chinese attack of India in October 1962. Dalvi's book was based supposedly on his official report about the Sino-Indian war, when he and many other Indian soldiers were arrested by the Red Army.

I read the book later and was shocked to know that so many elementary things regarding high altitude war were unknown to authorities. Example: *Khadi* blankets were supplied to soldiers. There was no supply of essential stationery items. Messages were written by charcoal on large sized *chapatis* (handmade bread) and sent to adjacent camps. What a small innovation this was! The Chinese soldiers were on the other side of a small river, wrote Dalvi. They used to address Indian soldiers in Hindi, sarcastically telling them to look at themselves and compare them with the Chinese soldiers. Dalvi wrote that if a Chinese soldier was caught, the arrested person would have to be taken to Delhi for interrogation.

However, we know that during those years Indian Army's war preparedness was not adequate. It was also not a priority item on the agenda. In fact, Gandhiji desired to disband the Army. Many developing countries including China accepted the peace keeping *Panchasheel* initiative of Nehru. There was the '*Hindi-Chini Bhai Bhai*' warmth in Indo-Chinese relations. Chinese Prime Minister Zhou Enlai visited India at least thrice as gestures of good will. Nehru was more shocked than angered by the Chinese aggression. At the same time, there were several hints given by China on border-related issues, which went unnoticed.[1]

Brigadier Dalvi's powerful and direct style of delivery influenced me very much. We spent long hours during the evenings when he spoke at length about the politics of international relations. We became friends, despite the difference in our ages.

The course went off greatly to my satisfaction. The sessions were engaging. That was the first time that I got exposed to many dimensions about which I did not know much. I realized that I was living in a closed environment, unaware of so many things happening outside Narendrapur. I thought that an unexplored new world was there for me to explore. I developed friendship with many participants.

My reading was reasonably wide but scattered, which included literature, political and economic thoughts, art and culture. I realized that I would have to focus on certain specific areas of learning relating to Economics in a broad sense. Large numbers of books were suggested. I read many of them after returning from the seminar. That profusely helped to widen and deepen my understanding. I made a number of friends, both with the faculty members as well as participants. I maintained postal correspondence with some of them. That was not the IT age. We had to write letters and I was not too bad a letter writer.

The following year, I took part in a program organized by LSPTD in Grand Hotel, Calcutta. In that seminar, my proposal to include Environmental Awareness in school curriculum was accepted. Masani fully supported the idea. This is was the first time that the subject of environment was accorded recognition in a forum.

Returning to Narendrapur, I realized, perhaps it was time to make a move. I had already thought about it deeply. There was some emotional engineering done to me to think about the prospect of my joining the Ramakrishna order as a monk. I received both direct and indirect hints from competent quarters.

That pushed me into thinking about 'What should I do with my life?'

Did someone micro manage our life? Did the belief in a super power work as a psychological relief? Why then were so many people suffering? Why do thousands have to die every year in natural disasters? Why were there devastating wars? Why Almighty did not help those suffering people? What bad deed so many people do in their past life? I know that believers would laugh at my ignorance. Let them.

I did some careful thinking about what I should do with my one small life. The book, 'What Should I Do with My Life' by Po Bronson,[2] based on large number of interviews of real life people answering this critical question was not published then. I did not get a direct reference point to check how people thought about what to do in life.

One day I was taking a class. Suddenly the thought came to mind like a powerful wave. I completed the class, went back to my hostel, applied for a few days leave, packed my bags and arrived at Howrah station. All that happened in a way as if it was planned, it was not so. I reached there as if getting pushed from inside. I was in a kind of a mild trance.

After reaching Howrah station, I realized that I did not know where to go. I heard someone buying a ticket for Puri. Thus prompted, I also bought a ticket to Puri. What about the reservation for my sleeper berth? It was one full night's journey. I need a berth to sleep.

To cut a long story short, an unknown person, who looked like a tout, came forward to help me with my reservation without any service charge. We remained friends for a long time. There are good souls among common people, we cannot always identify them.

Reaching Puri in the morning, I waited for a particular *Panda*, a priest who helped people to go to the Jagannath Temple for darshan and

Puja. I got to know him from my previous trip when we came to Puri with students under the leadership of Parameshwer da. Some of these *Panda* families maintain records of the visiting person's ancestral history. During my previous visit, I came across this *Panda*, Ram babu, who gave me details of my family's names and addresses. My grandfather and family once visited Puri. Ram babu's ancestors maintained records. I was surprised and ran through the documents. Yes, our family details and addresses were there. I thought that an empirical research should be conducted about such record keeping, their methods used and the authenticity of the records per say.

Ram babu took me to a modest but clean hotel near Swargadwar. We had stayed in a small building the previous time. The building was so uniquely constructed that the sea was visible from every room from the three sides facing the sea. The hotel was clean and simple. Food was also available. I spent three days alone on the beach, amidst the rolling sounds of waves being crushed. During the day, the Sun up in the sky was like a huge ball of fire and mad e the sand on the beach blistering hot. At night, it was very pleasant. The long waves showed glimmer of light as they contained phosphorus fluorescents. The rolling sound amidst slightly bright lights on the rolling waves created a heavenly experience. The sky above was clear with zillions of stars twinkling. The color of the sky was midnight blue. Rich and successful people wore suits of that color.

My mind was active during those days. I was thinking in a systematic way, organizing pluses and minuses of various career options.

Thinking about carccr options, the available opportunities in the country during this that time the late 1960s and early 1970s – were meager. With just a Master's in Economics, what great career could I make? My readings might have covered several areas but those were not of much use for entering the world of a career. I was neither a chartered accountant, engineer nor doctor, the preferred career options, which were popular and market-friendly. I had no other professional expertise as well. I considered applying for admission in the MBA course run by Indian Institute of Management, Calcutta, established in 1961. The institute, located initially at Emerald Bower campus, was just next to our Department of Economics, Calcutta University. But how could I pay the fees of the program and manage other expenses? No educational loan was available during that time.

Thoughts like those made my mind heavy. To break away from such thoughts, I decided to pay a visit to the famous Konark temple for the second time. The first time I went was with a trip organized for school students and some teachers by Parameshwer da. The journey was horrendous. The private vehicle some of us hired was in a dilapidated condition. It broke down a number of times. We felt relieved once we were able to reach by spending almost double the time. The exquisite Sun Temple was built during 13th century, sculpted beautifully from one solid rock in the form of a giant chariot.

Thinking about the people who built the gorgeous temple my mind traveled backward on time. The tour around the temple made my mind relaxed. I had made my decision. Well, almost!

What Should I Do in Life?

*It is meal time again. Do we eat more when we fly long distance? In any case,
it breaks the monotony. Some airlines are parsimonious. In 1987, American
Airlines saved $ 40,000 by giving one less olive in each salad served in first class.*

After returning from Puri, I decided to re-visit my decision. The
straightforward question was what should I do in my life? Because
of my specific background, my approach to life would be to try to make
my destiny in my own way, if I may say so. These are in generics. What
is the specific area in which I will spend and devote my living days on
this planet?

I used to walk on the terrace of my hostel building alone at night. I
thought about several topics and did some follow up readings. I thought
that I should discuss with some experts. But I observed that even
experts or specialized persons do have a position already taken. They
usually do not add on. Their specialization, knowledge and skill sets are
compartmentalized. They hardly possess a holistic approach. They have
not converted their knowledge into wisdom, or wisdom into insight. It
is difficult to find such insightful persons.

I have no problem with these so-called experts. I know a goldsmith
would not be able to make something a carpenter could do. The point
here is that finding a person with a holistic perception or a comprehensive
and insightful view about life in general and the ways of leading life in
particular is very rare. At the same time, the fact is that many issues do
overlap in life. Therefore, I have to find my own answer.

I am not making a big issue about it. I am just trying to narrate how I
did pass through this process of decision-making. I am a humble person

with a humble background. I just wanted to know, find my answer after running through a few options. It is my one simple life. Already more than a quarter century has been lived in getting ready for the next big round. I short-listed three specific options where from I would now choose one and move fast to make it a success.

One theoretical option, which I had already ruled out, was joining active politics. I know I am not an activist type. I read quite some books about Left ideologies. I am fully aware of the need for a home grown left of the center ideology for India; the adopted or copied models from abroad cannot work here. In any case, the option of being a political activist was not for me.

The second option, in a distinct contrast to the former was relating to joining the Ramakrishna order as a monk.

I am not a natural devotee. My head does not easily bend for a bow to a deity, or to a person. I do not believe or disbelieve in the existence of God or that God micro manages our lives. I know believing in God makes life easy and simple. Surrendering to God makes life easier. It gives huge amount of psychological relief.

I did some humble reading of our scriptures and discussed with several knowledgeable persons including senior monks. As a student of Ramakrishna Mission, I had to take a course on Indian Culture, taught by erudite monks – they are all believers. I took the course with seriousness. I know that the Bhagavad Gita has relevant learning for all. Under our Indian Culture course, the Epics, the Mahabharata and the Ramayana and the essences of certain *Upanishads* like *Katha Upanishad* were discussed. I also did some follow up readings. Still today, I do read some of the *Upanishads*, written so lucidly by Bada Maharaj. He presented to me several of his books with his signed autograph. They are my great treasures. The *Upanishads* are exquisitely written poems, or hymns. Incidentally, Swami Vivekananda said that when some thousands of years ago our *Rishis* had been writing those beautiful verses, Westerners were painting their body blue and were roaming in the forest!

When I was in 10th standard, I was greatly impressed and influenced by Christian hymns sung so magnificently in a church. I took a course on the Bible. Jesus' crucifixion pained me a lot. It does even today. I was about to become a Christian. However, it did not happen. News came in the press about some unlawful activities carried out by some persons in the church premises.

I did visit a number of so-called miracle makers, some *sadhus* and *fakirs* of the time. I personally saw several renowned people visited those so-called miracle makers. I went to one such fortuneteller in North 24 Parganas. He used to sit inside a room with the door shut. There was some thuggish looking assistants outside; one of them read the name and age of the person in front of the closed door. The *Baba* would shout something from inside. Another assistant would later explain to the concerned client the details and give some so-called Ayurvedic medicine, if required. Donations were most welcome.

I went there with a friend. We played a trick. When my turn came, I gave the name of a well-known politician. *Baba* went on giving his scripted message for a prospective young person. The assistant realized the trick and shouted for the bouncers. We ran fast to safety and laughed our lungs out. The session with Babas was shut that day.

There were some well-known astrologers and one Bhrigu muni in Murshidabad, West Bengal. I went to him. I wanted to know if there was a past life, who I was in my past life. Bhrigu muni advised me to come another day. I sat on planchettes a number of times. I was not impressed. I lived with my questions. Brain Weiss wrote his first book on past life regression much later – in 1988.[1,2] Even after reading his book on past life regression in later years, my questions remain unanswered.

The fundamental question of life and death, and that of God's existence or non-existence, the process of our being born, living a life and dying at the end is complex. Usually the common people accepts life as God given. They do not sit on judgment. In good times, they praise their God, in bad times they cry for help. They pray to their God for material wellbeing, recovery from diseases, passing exams, getting a good job, for marriage and for begetting children. This was known as 'Cupboard Love' for God, we read about it in our Intermediate classes. They go to the monks, astrologers, God men and accept their dictates or sermons. The rich do pujas and rituals by spending huge amounts of money and the poor also try their best even by borrowing money. At the end, they think God will take care of their problems. Look at the world at large – sufferings, problems and disasters, are all there aplenty across the globe – and growing at exponential rate.

It is not that the human beings alone live on planet Earth. There are many other 'beings' like the countless animals, creatures of all kind, even the plants and innumerable micro-organisms are all born, live a life of their own and eventually die under the natural process. This process of life or death of all beings – all of them from micro-organisms to plants to animals to humans from generations after generations on this tiny planet called Earth – have been going on from the day 'life' was initially formed. What if there are aliens in other planets many light years away, where life was formed billions of years ago? Is this not a statistical probability?

I have used the word 'formed' consciously, so as not to confuse with the word 'created', which would imply that somebody Super, i.e. God, might have created the world. Believers of course are there in millions. Their life is relaxed as they can leave their problems to their God.

These questions come to my mind from the 'Existential' philosophy of life, which appealed to me albeit up to a point, as a rational human being. I knew that these questions could not be answered in a linear or one-dimensional way.

These are the issues, which were discussed by the 'Existentialist' philosophers from Kierkegaard to Dostoyevsky, to Nietzsche, to my once favorite Jean Paul Sartre. It was Sartre, who wrote that "…existence precedes essence", meaning that individuals are for individuals and that "…they are independently acting and are responsible, conscious beings…". Sartre declined to accept the Nobel Memorial Prize in 1964 because he was not willing to be an 'institution', which he thought he would be if he had accepted the Nobel decoration.[3] He wanted to remain as an individual. I do appreciate such a stand in life. Ironically, by declining the Nobel, Sartre made himself unique and famous, i.e. an institution. He just missed the money.

I read and reread 'The Stranger' by Albert Camus. While some critics tagged him as 'Existentialist', he himself said he was not. After he wrote,

'*The Myth of Sisyphus*', some critics wrote that he was an advocate of 'Absurdism'. Camus wrote succinctly, "… I could see that it makes little difference whether one dies at the age of thirty or threescore and ten – since, in either case, other men will continue living, the world will go on as before. Also, whether I died now or forty years hence, this business of dying had to be got through, inevitably."[4] Right!

My thinking those days moved with both Existentialism and Absurdism for the time being. I contemplated over those interesting thoughts. I discussed with some of my teachers and senior monks. Soon I realized that looking East wards – to our own rich philosophical thoughts – gives us a variety of options, whether you are a believer, an atheist or an agnostic.

From my childhood, I had seen death from the ringside, death of my grandmother, mother, younger brother, my father and my sister. I have seen people dying in political violence, in riots, at the time of flood and drought. We have seen massive deaths in history, during the two World Wars and many wars thereafter. There was not a decade without any major war, killing large number of people. Death has been historically phenomenal. Are such deadly things also micro-managed by some 'Super' entity?

It was my privilege to come across some monks, who definitely attained considerable degree of sublimity and serenity as well as wisdom and insight; their presence brings mental peace and comfort. They are the genuine monks, who have seriously tried to renounce worldly life and devoted their lives for seeking 'moksha', simultaneously working for the good of the people. They have walked on the razor's edge; it is not easy to follow such a difficult path, unless you have your faith and believe in God, their God. They are wonderful people, who have sacrificed their life to serve the cause of humanity.

I am not a believer; I also am not an atheist. An atheist has negative faith; perhaps, non-faith, if I may call it so. I am comfortable in thinking that I am an agnostic by choice. Metaphorically, if 'Godot', not exactly in the Samuel Beckettian sense[5], arrives today or tomorrow, and I realize His being here, I shall welcome HIM.

Under the circumstances, I decided to use my humble existence in pursuing a professional career, doing Economics and related research, lead my life with a strong sense of principle and values, and try to help people in every possible way that I can without any publicity, demonstration or advertisement. At the same time, I must try to maintain distinctiveness without pride, in my own humble way. I should live a life without demonstrative consumerism, but with reasonable comfort. I should be able to take proper care of my wife, child or children, my close folks and relatives and friends. I should be able to take care of those who would come to me. I would not need any diamond for my breakfast. I would try to bring a smile to a sad face that actually lit up with happiness when helped. I would try to ensure the sustenance of their happiness. I would try to hold some hands that need holding. I should sincerely strive to explore the horizon of knowledge, transcend it to wisdom and further to insight. I should be able seriously practice the virtue of *'Aparigrah'* (detachment, a rough translation).

Yes, life itself is a celebration. It is not denial of certain things. It has to be lived in full, yet avoiding conspicuous consumption. I want to see seasons changing from summer to rainy days, freshening up of the trees, which bring a gloss on the green leaves. The crown of the trees and plants look so green and lively after the break of the monsoon; they celebrate life. They dance with joy. I want to see beautiful autumn leaves with fiery colors on trees and on the ground in Virginia. I would like to enjoy a long 'fall foliage' drive with my folks on the roads of Michigan's Gold Coast. I would like to see the golden hues covered in the morning of Kangchenjunga. I want to look at the blue sky with floating clouds.

I would like to sit on the edge of the chair, work hard in my professional life and try to add value. Sure, I would like to move up in my profession, leave a mark by my honest, sincere and intelligent hard work. I want to come home to see the smiling faces of my wife and child/children; I would like to sit on the ground with them and have a relaxed time together. I should be able to enjoy small and beautiful things of life. I intend to keep my home open to my friends and relatives. I would like to fly like the Phoenix to live my life.

When we grow biologically old, I would like to sit with my best friend, my wife, and watch the day changing in the twilight glow. We would like to see the sad and soft colorful sky gradually enveloping into darkness. We would look at the night sky and watch the stars and stars and stars, enjoy the soothing cool wind comforting our limbs. Yes, I would like to meet my God, if I feel his presence in my mind. Then, time comes for me take part in the ultimate celebration of life – death, and merge with nature. I go back where from I have come.

Once I made up my mind, I knew that my time to leave Narendrapur had come. I wrote to J.P. Naik, the educationist, Chairman, ICSSR, New Delhi. Initially, the ICSSR office was in the IIPS building. We were also staying in the IIPS hostel for one of our research methodology courses. Since we were taking part in the ICSSR sponsored course, I had an opportunity to know J.P. Naik.

He advised me to apply to ICSSR for a research fellowship. Eventually, a reputed economist approved my project proposal, and I received the 'pay protection' research fellowship of ICSSR, which was introduced in the same year.

Incidentally, the then well known *Bhrigu Muni* of Murshdabad district, West Bengal made a number of predictions about my present life. One was that I would get '*Raj Dware Arthaprapti, Taddwara Veda Avhash*'. Interpreting it in today's language, he said, that I would receive scholarship from government and do research work. Of course, while discussing with him I had mentioned that I had applied for a scholarship. When I think about it, it comes to my mind that was he so smart to catch the point of scholarship and made his prediction. How could he 'predict' this one right? Well, I have no answer.

I resigned from the school and left Narendrapur on the last week of December 1972. A long chapter of my life – my growing up years, precisely 13 years, ended.

Thank you for everything, my dear Narendrapur!

CHAPTER

19

One Decision, Millions Suffer

I settled down on my seat and thought about the waves of refugees who moved in search of a safe destination. How many of us moved out from the eastern side of Bengal?

There have been unpredictable and immeasurable changes in the socio-economic and political life in West Bengal since Independence, accompanied by the partition of India. The partition resulted in steady inflow of refugee migrants from East Pakistan into West Bengal.

The geographical area of West Bengal is 89,000 sq km, which obviously remains a constant. It is just 2.7% of India's total area. But the population has been increasing rapidly, from 23.2 million in 1941 to 91.3 million in 2011, almost by four times. The population of West Bengal in 2011 was as high as 8% of India's population. This high population created pressure on the limited area of land. The density of population moved up sharply from 264 per sq km in 1941 to 1,028 in 2011 – by almost four times. Apart from the natural growth of population, which was not too high in West Bengal, the important contribution to growth came from migration of refugee population over the years from East Bengal, rechristened Bangladesh since 1971.

Look at Karnataka in contrast – the state's area is 192,000 sq km, more than double that of West Bengal. Its population rose from 26.3 million in 1951 (slightly more than West Bengal's) to 61 million in 2011 (about 67% of West Bengal's). The density in 2011 was 320 per sq km, little more than one third of West Bengal's.

Various estimates have been made about the migration and infiltration of people from East Pakistan/ Bangladesh regularly to West

Bengal, which has been going on since 1946 until 1991 in phases. Actually, illegal migrants do arrive even today crossing the long border.

How many people have moved from East Pakistan, now Bangladesh, to India since the partition of Bengal? It is not easy to answer. There is no definite count available.

According to 1951 Census of Displaced Persons, 7.2 million Muslims went to West Pakistan from India immediately after the partition, while 7.3 million Hindu and Sikh population moved as refugees from West Pakistan to India. Again, out of these 14.5 million, about 11.2 million or 78 % displaced persons were on the western side. About 6.5 million Muslims went to West Pakistan from India; and 4.7 million Hindus moved from West Pakistan to India.

From the remaining 3.3 million, 2.6 million or 26.6% Hindus migrated from East Pakistan to India and only 0.7 million Muslims from India to East Pakistan. These are the estimated numbers of refugees till 1951, i.e., 40 months from the time of partition.

Looking at West Bengal, we find an estimate of the Government of West Bengal, which indicates that 4.45 million refugees have entered West Bengal during 1946–1970, a period of 25 years.[1]

During the 1950s and 1960s, there were several spurts in people from East Pakistan entering West Bengal. During the Independence War of Bangladesh, 1971, according to United Nations High Commissioner for Refugees (UNHCR) estimate, 10 million people crossed the border and arrived in West Bengal. It was as if floodwater was gushing out after the dam gate was opened. Many political leaders of the then East Pakistan and teachers from schools to universities were staying in Calcutta. Three teachers also stayed in Narendrapur and taught in our school.

From Ramakrishna Mission, Narendrapur, we organized a relief camp somewhere at Bongaon or Basirhat, North 24 Parganas. It was located near a small river; on the eastern side was East Pakistan and West Bengal on the western side. Two boats were placed one after the other to build a make shift bridge. I personally witnessed and photographed the flow of people entering our side, day and night for several days. It was a difficult task to feed them. We served *khichari,* a balanced meal of rice, pulse and vegetables twice a day.

Many important persons visited that camp. I saw many leaders from both sides visited the camp. They were accompanied by large number of companions. They created a mess in the name of visiting the distressed people. They were busy photographing themselves with some refugees and interviewed by the Press. They left after saying empty words of sympathy and promise of help.

I remember Prince Aga Khan's visit. He was different. He took the trouble of talking to a large number of people in the camp. A correspondent from All India Radio was translating for him. He watched for some time the distribution of milk. We used to give one mug of milk for one kid per day. It was not possible to verify whether the person in the queue had kids or not. Aga Khan was watching the queue for quite some time asking people about their kids, shaking his head in pain and sadness. I did some brief explanation to him. I personally followed his visit. I realized that his concern for the refugees was genuine. He asked about Ramakrishna Mission, details about how we were running the camp and how we got funds. Sure, he did announce a large amount of grant the next day.

We could hear the sound of firing; watch the burning of houses at night on the East Pakistan side. When India declared the war, the Indian Army entered East Pakistan and the killing of people stopped in that area, which was clearly visible from our side. Returning to Narendrapur, I did display my photographs in our school premises.

Eventually, the war ended on December 16, 1971 when Lt Gen Niazi signed the surrender document and handed it over to Lt Gen Jagjit Arora; and an Independent Bangladesh was born on December 16, 1971.

Out of over 10 million people who entered India at the time of the war, a small number of Muslim population, about 62,000, went back home to their newly Independent country Bangladesh. However, majority of the Hindu population, about 10 million stayed on. They were the new refugees added to the population of West Bengal. It was not possible to count the exact numbers.

The long U-shaped border of 4,096 kms makes it easy for people from Bangladesh to cross the border and enter India, which, in their perception, is a land of better opportunities. Besides, it is common knowledge that ruling political parties have been helping the migrant population directly or indirectly, say by issuing them ration cards and entering their names to the voters list to create a vote bank. These illegal migrants or regular infiltrators are not counted as refugees.

Various estimates have been made about the migration or infiltration of people from East Pakistan/ Bangladesh regularly to West Bengal, which has been going on since 1946 till 1991 in phases. According to an estimate[2], 13 to 14 million people entered India from Bangladesh during 1971 through 1991. While some of these people have gone to neighboring states, majority of them have settled in West Bengal. Adding the number of 4.45 million refugees who entered India during 1946 to 1970 to the above mentioned number of 13to 14 million, the total numbers of entrants becomes as large as 19 million.

However, according to UNHCR and other sources[2] the total number of refugees due to partition of India is 14 million. Besides, the war of Independence of Bangladesh unleashed 10 million refugees. It is difficult to verify the consistency of these estimates.

The number of 14 million has been used in yet another estimate. Using data originating from UNHCR, NATO, Migration Policy Institute, Refugees International, US State Department and Press reports, *The Economist*, May 28, 2016, confirmed that 14 million people moved as refugees in to India.[3]

However, the breakdown of this estimate is not available. Hindu refugee migrants arrived in batches. The first batch of arrivals was immediately after partition. Then during the 1950s and 1960s, several waves of people arrived due to certain political or military exigencies. Thereafter arrived the wave of refugee migrants at the time of the War of Independence of Bangladesh in 1971, estimated at about 10 million.

Thus, the total number of refugees, who came in to India from Bangladesh, according to my estimate, would be around 20 million plus. Largely, we can use this number, 20 million, to be the estimated number of refugees who have moved into India after 1947.

What I intend to highlight here is that the partition made a great paradigm shift in the Bengali society because of this huge 20 million migrant of population. They caused immense pressure on the small area of West Bengal as well as on its demography, socio-economic and political life. At the same time, those people have also contributed to the Bengali society in many areas like enhancing the importance of education, political awareness and cultural interchange. It is difficult to make a cost benefit analysis of this historic event, the partition.

The other side of the picture would have to be considered from the point of view of the Muslim population. Immediately before the partition, the Muslim population in undivided Bengal, under the influence of their leaders, desired to have their own State. They were in favor of the partition of Bengal. That was largely because they did not get sufficient opportunity for growth and development in Bengal. In the field of education, health and hygiene as well as employment, the Muslim community's participation was low.

The relationship between the Hindu and Muslim community was two – dimensional. On the one plain, they were living peacefully together. Yet it was a reality that the standard of living, level of education, health and hygiene and occupational status of the Muslim community in general was lower than those of the Hindus. It was true that there were well-settled, rich and aristocratic Muslims, but they were small in number. Despite long centuries of Muslim rule, the overall standards of living of the community had not improved. Why it has not happened is long story.

Simply put, the discrimination in terms of castes, creeds and religion practiced by the dominating Hindus was one of the causes. This discrimination did not spare even the large number of people belonging to the so-called lower caste people. In fact, thousands of so-called lower caste Hindus abandoned their religion and became Muslims or Christian. All first generation Muslim and Christian population originally belonged to the Hindu mainstream of life in India. Because of this torture, humiliation, discrimination even in the recent time, in 1956, Baba Saheb Ambedkar left Hindu religion along with his followers and formed the Neo – Buddhist class.

What I also intend to point out here is that because of the partition and the formation of Independent Bangladesh, there are 170 million people presently living in Bangladesh, out of which 85% are Muslims about 13 to 14% Hindus and 1to 2% belong to other religions. In Bangladesh, Muslim people are employed in government, legislature, judiciary, military services, public and private sector industries, in education, art, culture and literature i.e., in every sector of the economy and society. They are the majority with small share of jobs going to the minority population. Simply put, the partition of Bengal has benefited the Muslim people in Bangladesh in many ways. They now have their own State, with a distinctive Muslim majority. They run their own affairs.

Behind this success story lays the suffering of 20 million to 24 million Hindu refugees, who had to rush out from their own home during partition and thereafter.

Today Bangladesh is a unique example of improving its social indicators though they are yet to experience high level of per capita GDP on PPP basis, $3,900 compared to $6,700 of India in 2016.[4]

Running through Bangladesh Progress Report, 2015[5], we get a clear picture of significant improvement in various socio-economic parameters relating to millennium development goals of the United Nations.

Besides, there has been rapid progress in publications in Bengali language in Bangladesh in various subjects including literature, fiction and non-fiction as well as technical books. The historic Language Movement that culminated on February 21, 1952 raised the role and status of Bengali as the official language of the erstwhile East Bengal, now Bangladesh. The contribution of the young people for their love of the language has been written in history in golden letters. UNESCO has declared February 21 as the International Mother Language Day.

Presently, about 250 million people in Bangladesh and West Bengal and some adjacent states speak Bengali. It is a recognized language in the UN systems. There has been increasing cultural exchange between West Bengal and Bangladesh in literature, music and movies including people-to-people exchange.

To conclude this chapter, the so-called refugees did not remain as 'refugees' in West Bengal. They were not a perpetual burden. They have contributed not only to the State's economic growth, but also to the socio-political and cultural arena. They have moved up the ladders of life and established themselves as proud citizens of India. The heroic initiative of their children in facing challenges of life, using the platform of education, brought in a huge positive impact on the overall socio-economic canvas of West Bengal.

CHAPTER
20

Political 'Governance' in Bengal

Lights are dim inside. The flight is racing forward. Looking at the flight map on the screen, I thought what a marvel of aviation technology! We will reach Mumbai from New York in just 16 hours. How many months would a ship have taken to cover this distance hundred years ago? Yet we get impatient.

I have grown up hearing that Bengalis love 'politics'. It is true. Do they also love 'politicking'?

A quick study of West Bengal's assembly election shows that the Indian National Congress (INC) formed, naturally so, the first government immediately after Independence. INC got a high 63% seats in the first ever assembly election in 1951. Its share of seats came down to 60.3% in 1956. Their share slightly moved up to 62.3% in 1962, the year of the Chinese aggression. Thereafter, INC's share of seats steadily came down to 45% in 1967, further to 19.6% in 1969 and just 6.8% in 1977. In 1987, its share slightly improved to 13.6%; further to 14.6% in 1991. Then INC virtually disappeared from the scene; its share came down to a meager 1.4% in 2011 assembly election. Meanwhile, a group led by Mamata Banerjee, a firebrand and street-smart politician, broke out from INC and formed Trinamool Congress on January 1, 1998.

On the other side, the undivided Communist Party of India (CPI), which eventually adopted the parliamentary democracy abandoning the 'revolutionary' path, got 11.8% share of seats in the assembly election of 1951, moved up its seat share to 19.8% in 1962. The CPI was divided in 1962 as an aftermath of the Chinese aggression, and the Communist Party of India-Marxist, CPI (M) was formed. The CPI existed as a small party. The share of seats of CPI (M) in assembly election was as high as 60.5% in 1977, moved up to 63.6% in 1987, but reduced to about 60% in 2006, and came down drastically to 13.6% in 2011.

Other left parties, as many as 15 of them in 2011, also passed through vicissitudes; from 5.5% seats share in 1951 to a high 28.6% in 1969, 24.8% in 2006, and just 6.1% in 2011. The CPI has been marginalized; its share of seats was a meager 0.7% in 2011.

The large number of Left parties apart from CPI (M), as many as 17 Left parties in West Bengal in 2011, tells its own story of Bengal politics, or even 'politicking'. In 1973, Fidel Castro had a two-hour stop over at Dumdum Airport, now called Netaji Subash Airport. Jyoti Basu and some others met him. They discussed about Indian and Bengal politics. On hearing that there were a large number of communist parties, a surprised Fidel commented, '17 communist parties'!

Largely, the informed people know about Communist or Socialist ideologies. Yet what are such minute and defining issues that there has to be 17 Left parties? Actually, many of these parties are single leader parties, or dominated by a couple of leaders in a couple of constituencies where they have some influence due to some historical reasons. The small party leaders stake their claim as ministers in the new the Government after an election. It is not ideology; it is self interest – getting a slot in the cabinet – is the issue. To my mind, this is 'politicking'.

During the long period of 65 years of assembly election, several changes have happened in West Bengal's political scene. For obvious reasons, the partitioned-affected refugee population sided with the undivided CPI in the beginning, and subsequently with CPI (M) as well as other left parties in their clusters of influence.

A group led by Ajoy Mukherjee, a veteran Congressman, moved away from INC and formed Bangla Congress. This was a turning point of Bengal politics. The first United Front (UF) Government was formed with the support of Bangla Congress on March 1, 1967. Ajoy Mukherjee was the Chief Minister and Comrade Jyoti Basu was the Deputy Chief Minister in the newly formed first U F government. The new Government announced an 18-point program. That was a critical time because of acute food shortage. However, there were differences of opinion among the constituent parties of the first UF government.

It failed to sustain majority and was dismissed by the Governor at the instruction of the INC led Central Government on November 21, 1967. This led to a huge unrest in Bengal. Processions, angry outbursts, street corner meetings and *gheraos* in offices went on merrily. The Left front called a 48-hour Bengal *bandh*, which was successful.

INC, with the Chief Ministership of Dr. Prafulla Chandra Ghosh, formed a minority government for just 90 days. Eventually, Dr. Ghosh had to resign and President's rule was imposed in West Bengal during 1968–69. This again caused huge unrest on the streets of Calcutta. Processions, meetings, agitations and strikes became a part of Calcutta's daily life.

Dr. Ghosh was Chief Minister three times, each for a short duration. He was an idiosyncratic person, earnestly following the Gandhian style of living, a confirmed bachelor, wearing *khadi* clothes, eating simple food and living a spartan life. He was an example of those simple living but high thinking idealistic types.

He had many fascinating stories to tell. He would always speak in the dialect version of Bengali as spoken in East Bengal. The original inhabitants of West Bengal called the people, who came from East Bengal *Bangals* in a somewhat unwelcome way. The *Bangals* in turn returned the ridicule by calling people of West Bengal as *Ghotis*. Trying to get the etymology of *Ghoti* would lead us nowhere. Yet these two terms are widely used in Bengal even today. *Bangals* spoke with heavy and emphatic accent and at high decibels, which was different from the Bengali spoken by the educated people of Calcutta.

Dr. Ghosh used to visit Bada Maharaj occasionally. On one occasion when Bada Maharaj was in Ramakrishna Mission Seva Pratisthan for treatment, Dr. Ghosh came to visit him and I was there. Bada Maharaj got up from his bed and sat in a half-inclined position with a smile on his face. We knew that we would have great time now. After courtesy talk, Dr. Ghosh returned to his usual self. Seeing me present, he was enthused. He got young company. He asked me about my background. Bada Maharaj told him about me. He started his immensely enjoyable chat with his interpretation of food values and nutrition of very simple and cheap food stuff as was consumed by common people.

The nutritional quality of puffed rice, soaked *channa*, common leafy vegetables and *gur* were explained superbly. He was a scientist himself. His narration in the *Bangal* dialect, mixed with scientific terms as well as humor and wit, made us roar with laughter.

The assembly election was held in 1969; for the first time CPI (M) got the largest party status with 28.6% seat share. CPI got 10.7 %. All other heterogeneous left parties also got as high as 28.6%. The share of seats of all left parties together was as high as almost 68%. INC's share of seats was reduced to 19.6%. Thus, the second UF government was formed in West Bengal in 1969–70 for one year and 155 days again with Ajoy Mukherjee as CM and Jyoti Basu as Deputy CM. [1]

There was great enthusiasm of people at large. Literally, millions gathered in the *Maidan*, Dalhousie Square, the down town of Calcutta, now called BBD Bagh, to hear Jyoti Basu and other senior leaders of the UF. The Raj Bhavan gates were forced opened. Thousands of people rushed into the palatial residence of the Governor, which was the office and residence of the Governor General of British India till 1911 when Calcutta was the capital of British India. People damaged the beautiful garden. I think that rushing to the Raj Bhavan was an impulsive event. It was more of a sudden emotional upsurge. The crowd disappeared within a few hours.

The problem for the second UF government was more or less the same as earlier. There was strong difference of opinion among the constituent parties; there were too many of them. The Government had to resign on July 30, 1970. Again, President's Rule was imposed on July 30, 1970 for the fourth time for 215 days.

The formation of governments by Left parties and President's rule went on alternating frequently. As a result, development works became a victim. What great initiatives could be taken under such circumstances? Ajoy Mukherjee led yet another UF Government, which came to office for the third time, on April 2, 1971 just for 84 days, immediately followed by another round of President's Rule for268 days!

Subsequently, the INC government led by Siddharth Shankar Ray took office on March 20, 1972: it ruled West Bengal for the full term of five years until April 30, 1977. Again for a short period of 51 days

President's Rule – the fourth one – was imposed on April 30, 1977, ending the musical chair contest between the democratically elected government's rule and the President's Rule.

The Naxalite movement raised its head during that time. In addition, during this period industrial unrest started growing, followed by flight of capital. In sum, a massive turmoil and churning in the socio-political life moved like a volcanic eruption, destroying the peace and harmony in public life, to say the least about developmental activities.

As is well known, CPI (M) had to suffer a split in 1967 when a certain leaders of the party formed a communist guerrilla group, inspired by the so-called revolutionary agrarian movement in Naxalbari in North Bengal under the leadership of Kanu Sanyal and Jongal Santhal. Thus, CPI (Marxist Leninist) was set up under the ideological inspiration from Comrade Mao Zedong, and under the local leadership of Charu Mazumdar and Saroj Dutta, who broke away from CPI (M) and formed CPI (ML) on April 22, 1969. In a mass meeting on in the *Maidan,* the formation of the new revolutionary party was announced. The new party abandoned the path of parliamentary democracy and adopted the path of armed revolution. Kanu Sanyal and Jongal Santhal, two leaders of Naxalbari agrarian movement also joined CPI (ML), making the 'Naxalite' synonymous to the new party's formal name.

The call for establishing a Marxist – Leninist Communist society had its appeal to the young Bengali people particularly college students. Many of them abandoned their studies, got emotionally charged, joined the party and over a period spread across the villages of West Bengal, and later to Bihar, UP and other neighboring states. They were dreaming to establish a Communist society in India. A massive unrest and violence were set in motion. The usually vibrant Calcutta life changed into scary and fearful one.

In 1971, Charu Mazumdar, the top leader of CPI (ML), gave a call for the 'annihilation line', i.e. assassinating the individual class enemy. Soon the new party was split, initially into two, later to several splinter groups. The original CPI (ML) was dissolved on July 31, 1972.

Using President's Rule in West Bengal, the 'Operation Steeplechase' was unleashed, killing thousands and arresting over 20,000 suspects and cadres, including senior leaders as well as many innocents.[2]

The Congress came to power in 1972 election led by Siddhartha Sankar Ray as already mentioned. The CPI (M) boycotted the assembly for five years till 1977, an absurd decision. The party accepted parliamentary democracy, yet the decision to boycott the assembly for five long years defied common sense.

The new Ray government took a very tough stance to handle Naxalites without any opposition. Chief Minister Siddhartha Sankar Ray pledged to 'solve' the Naxalite problem. There were reports almost every day in the daily newspapers that in an 'encounter' with the police so many Naxalite young persons were dead. It was a very sad period for West Bengal.

When we were doing a course in the Indian Statistical Institute, I distinctly remember shrieking sounds of a person, with repeated appeal 'do not kill me' coming from rear side of the institute in the middle of the night. The next morning we heard that a young boy was stabbed to death. On yet another occasion when we were walking from the hostel to the institute, a short distance of about one hundred meters, we saw the dead body of a young boy with the gunshot lying on the BT Road. The angelic face of the boy still haunts me.

Moving over to the country as a whole, INC used to rule the Central Government those days. The INC Government could not tolerate the formation of the government by the CPI (M) led governments. In fact, the first CPI (undivided)-led Government was formed in Kerala in 1957 under the leadership of Comrade EMS Namboodripad. The EMS Government introduced radical land and education reform measures. However, the existence of a Communist state in India, allegedly, was not acceptable to several powerful forces, at home and abroad. Eventually, President's Rule was imposed in 1959 in Kerala using the controversial article 356 of the Indian Constitution. The Central Government run by the Congress was allergic to the CPI/ CPI(M) rule in Kerala or Bengal.

With the formation of the UF Government with CPI (M) majority in 1977 began the end of a long spell of four short lived governments inter-spaced by four short spells of President's Rule in West Bengal during 1967–72. Siddharth Roy's full five-year rule (1972–77) was largely devoted to containing the Naxalite movement as explained later.

Such frequent changes of Government and imposition of President's Rule meant that hardly any developmental work was taken up during this period.

Besides, the decade of the 1960s began with the Chinese aggression in 1962, followed by the Indo-Pak war in 1965–66.

An intense social tension was going on in West Bengal since the late 1960s. The suspension of the UF Government in 1967, the disruption by the Naxalite movement, the growing violence in society in the name of political rivalry, almost daily processions clogging streets of Calcutta, strikes organized largely by trade unions belonging to the Left parties and the *gheraos* of company bosses went on unabated. As a result, there was steady flow of capital flight from West Bengal to other states in the country. No new large-scale investment did take place for a long period. Companies after companies shut down their operation.

Prime Minister Indira Gandhi declared a state of internal Emergency with effect from June 25, 1975, which was withdrawn on March 21, 1977, after a period of 21 months. This happened because of the verdict of the Allahabad High Court against Indira Gandhi's election. Reportedly, she had a deep sense of insecurity and felt that she might be overthrown as mentioned by Katherine Frank in her biography of Indira Gandhi.[3] The story of Emergency is well known.

On the day of the declaration of Emergency, I was in Mumbai. People rushed home. By noontime, the vibrant city wore a deserted look with not a soul around. Tapati was with me during those days. Seeing me home early, she was happy. I told her what had happened. There was only radio to get news. We had a small radio set. We turned on BBC as All India Radio would only give the official version. Many political leaders, college and university teachers and journalists with non-establishment views were arrested. The next morning, the *Indian Express* newspaper published a black bordered empty first page as a protest. We wondered whether we were going to have a dictatorial government in the country.

Jyoti Basu formed the United Left Front Government on June 21, 1977. Thus, began the era of 34 years of non-stop CPI (M) led left rule in West Bengal till 2011. It must be a world record that one group of Left party alliance under the leadership of CPI (M) continued to rule an Indian state winning seven assembly elections consecutively for 34 years at a stretch. However, the so-called stability eventually was metamorphosed into stagnation.

In the 1977 assembly election, CPI (M) along with all other left parties came to power with a huge popular mandate. CPI (M) got 63.6% seats in the assembly; all other left parties got almost 18% of seats; thus the Left front got almost 82% of seats. INC got just 6.8% seats, virtually washed out in the electoral politics. Perhaps, the ruthlessness of Siddharth Roy government in handling the Naxalites could have been one reasons for the rout of the Congress in the election.

During the historic long period of democratic power, from 1977 until 2011, the CPI (M)-led Government initiated several landmark works particularly in agriculture and rural development. The U F Government took up agriculture as their area of serious concern. Under its famous Operation (Ops) *Barga*, legal amendments were enacted to change the age-old relationship between landlords and *bargadars* (farm laborers who cultivate lands). The eviction of *bargadars* was made impossible under the amended law. Besides, a fair share of crops was guaranteed. In fact, no other state in India addressed any land reform related issues. Precisely, the Ops *Barga* of CPI (M) led UF Government made significant progress in three specific areas, namely, regulating share cropping pattern and redistributing ceiling-surplus land in ownership by introducing Land Ceiling Act as well as distributing home plots.

Empirical studies were carried out on the Ops *Barga*, and it was found that the volume of agricultural production, productivity, employment, income including fair distribution of income and better utilization of *barga* considerably improved initially. Ops *Barga* also improved irrigation facilities and land use pattern as well as the status of the farm laborers. As a result, over two million farm laborers benefited; complaints of starvation deaths and suicides were not heard of until recently.

However, gains in agriculture through the Ops *Barga*, initially improved for a number of years, and then plateaued out thereafter, decelerating the rate of improvement.

The next round of measures likes rural/ agricultural products marketing, training of the farm laborers for using new technology, development of entrepreneurial culture, cold chain, necessary infrastructure and all that were ignored. The simple point was that the farmer must get an appropriate return on investment in the farm. This point was not considered.

Besides, there was not even a serious discussion about making an effort towards solving the age-old, albeit serious structural problem regarding too much segregation and fragmentation of land and the high landmass to the population ratio, which was very high in West Bengal. Some lame effort might have been there on papers about trying to take up cooperative/ community type of farming but it was not pursued. Perhaps, an 'Amul' equivalent approach might have done something good in that regard.

The Naxalite phenomenon was accompanied with continuing political unrest, protests against the Congress government, aggressive trade unionism and closures of industries and flight of capital, growing unemployment and all that had been developing into a critical mass, gravitating into an enormous black hole. In a separate chapter, I have discussed the long de-industrialization in Bengal.

In the 2011 assembly election, the Trinamool Congress (TMC), which broke away from INC in 1998, obtained 184 seats, a percentage share of 62.6% of total seats of 294, and captured almost 39% of total votes polled. West Bengal Congress, a partner of TMC in 2011 election, got 42 seats, the combined share of seats of both the parties was as high as almost 226. Seats of CPI (M) came down sharply from 176 in 2006 to 42 seats in 2011; the combined Left Front got only 62 seats, a share of 21%. Contrast this pathetic result with the election of 2006 when the Left front received as high as 233 seats out of 294, a share of over 79% seats. In the 2006 election, the TMC got only 30 seats and the Congress 21.

Coming to the assembly election of 2016, the performance of TMC, despite continued wide spread political violence, was astounding. The

TMC again got a massive mandate; it received 211 seats alone (184 in 2011), with almost 72% share of assembly seats and almost 45% share of the popular votes polled.

In that election, the CPI (M) led Left parties partnered with their arch 'enemy', Congress. It was a contradiction of great height; the left front was fighting Congress in Kerala, while dancing together merrily in Bengal.

The supporters argued that the partnership was required for stopping the 'misrule' of TMC. However, the people voted for TMC; they ignored the 'misrule' and wide spread political violence. Out of 65.5 million voters in the assembly election of 2016, slightly over 80% cast their votes. There was a number of election related political violence in certain areas. But because of the presence and the alertness of the central forces and the supervision of the Election Commission of India, the election was reported to be successfully conducted.

In 2016 assembly election, the combined Left and Congress received 76 seats, with Left Front 32 and Congress even higher, 44 seats. The seat share of the Left was about 25.9% and CPI (M), with just 26 seats, got 8.8% seats. The share of valid votes polled was 44.9% for TMC with 211 seats, Left 25.9%, Congress 12.3% and Left Front plus Congress 38.2%. CPI (M)'s vote share came down almost by 10% from 29.6% in 2011 to 19.7% in 2016. The BJP emerged with three seats, a vote share of 10.7%.

The number of seat won by CPI(M) in the Lok Sabha election also came down sharply from 43 in 2004 to 15 in 2009, and further to just 9 in 2014, while those of TMC's improved from 2 to 19 to 34 during the same period. Similarly, the number of MPs of CPI (M) from West Bengal also came down from 26 in 2004 to just 2 in 2014, while those of TMC's increased from one to 34 during this period.[4] *Paribartan* in the number game!

Perhaps, a transformation in the political equation was in process. Meanwhile, the chaotic 'governance' is likely to continue. The overall socio-political environment in West Bengal has been witnessing massive increase in violence and unrest. It seems that a kind of anarchy has dawned on civil society. The situation is more or less the same in several other states of India. It might take a long time for this nightmare to pass.

CHAPTER 21

Making a Career

The price of one Boeing 777–9 aircraft is $ 426 million (2018), the highest end; that of the lowest one is $ 86 million for Boeing737–700. Because of this high price, direct cash transaction does not happen. Again, the margin of airlines business is low. Thus, the airlines business finance is very complex – sophisticated leases or debt financing schemes like secured lending or operating leasing, finance leasing, or a combination of them. There are other options as well.

There was a small hostel (popularly called *'mess'* in Bengal), in Dover Lane, Gariahat, South Calcutta, where I rented a room on the first floor. The location was convenient in every way. Gariahat is the heart of Calcutta's shopping center for *saris*, women's dresses and jewelry. Both commerce and culture mingle at Gariahat. From there you can reach anywhere in the city within a short time.

Talking of Dover Lane, the lovers of Indian Classical music would immediately recall The Dover Lane Music Conference (DLMC), an annual festival of Indian Classical Music, which was organized first by the local music lovers at Dover Lane in 1952. The office of the DLMC is still in Dover lane. The present venue of the Conference is Najrul Mancha, Ravindra Sarovar, located nearby. Most maestros of Indian Classical music have performed here.

My mind became blank after leaving Narendrapur. After leading a regulated campus life for 13 long years, suddenly I found myself sitting in a small and crampy room on the first floor of the mess. Looking through the only – tiny-window, my vision stuck to a shabby slum below. People were busy with their daily chores. I moved out of the room and melted into the crowded Gariahat crossing. The experience was like moving out of a solitary prison cell to a vibrant market place. I realized I should settle down to the new reality of my life.

My daily schedule was to go to the CMPO library to study for my research project, arrange a survey schedule for the project, meet top officials of the Ministry of Housing, Government of West Bengal and collect data and information. My supervisor, S.B. Mukherjee, was a nice, albeit a busy person. Spending a couple of hours with him even in a week was not always possible.

During this time, Tapati and I decided to get married. One afternoon, I approached my would be father-in-law, the formidable Tara Prasad Chakraborty, a former freedom fighter of repute as I have already mentioned. The government recognized his contribution as a freedom fighter by awarding him a *Tamrapatra*.

His family used to live in Banagram, Dhaka. His father, Mahim Chandra Chakraborty, was a 'Judge Pandit', appointed by the British government to teach British officers Indian Culture, Sanskrit and related topics. The family was highly esteemed. His elder brother was a double master's degree holder and was a teacher. Second brother was a doctor. He and his younger brother, Uma Prasad, joined the freedom movement.

Like many other freedom fighters, Marxism influenced him when he was in the British jail. By the time he was out, the country was about to be divided. He had to leave his lecturership from a college in East Bengal and move over to Calcutta. Initially, his family was staying at Bhabanipur. Subsequently, they moved to Bijaygarh, a large refugee colony in Jadavpur. He built a small house on a small plot of land. As a respected leader of the community, he took the initiative along with some of his friends to build several schools, both for the boys and girls, in the area where children of the locality got their education.

Being heartbroken because of the partition of the country, he decided to retire from active politics and got a job as an officer in the Refugee, Relief and Rehabilitation Ministry, Government of West Bengal. If the country was not partitioned and he would not have moved from his base, he might not have left active politics. It was not possible at his age to start afresh in Calcutta. His political understanding was superb. Several top Left party leaders used to discuss with him both ideological and real-life issues of politics.

Tapati is his first daughter. She also belonged to the Partition's Generation and struggled to come up in life and career. After doing graduation in Geography from Lady Brabourne College, Calcutta University, she completed her MA degree in Geography from University of Calcutta. She was employed in National Atlas and Thematic Mapping Organization, Government of India, as a young cartographer.

That was September 1973 in the afternoon, I went to see her father in his office in The Writers' Building, the seat of the Government. Tapati had informed him about our intention of getting married. Naturally, she told her parents about my background – that I had a bright future, but I had no material possession or family assets at all. I know no father of a daughter would agree to such a marriage.

All this should have been enough to discourage any father of a marriageable daughter. Under the circumstances, I had to tell him my story. Then, it was up to him to take a call. In any case, we were adults. We could also decide about ourselves. The point was that it would be gracious that the parents, relatives and friends also join the marriage. Thus, I went with an uncertain mind, but decided to talk straight and seek his permission for his daughter's hand.

I had visited The Writers' Building many times before. It is the secretariat of the State Government of West Bengal, India. It was constructed in several phases during the period 1777 through 1800, based on a design created by architect Thomas Lyon at the instance of Richard Barwell, member of the Council, during the governorship of Warren Hastings. The Writers' Building was leased out to the British East India Company for their junior officers, called writers. During later years, the Calcutta stock market was named after Thomas Lyon. Subsequently, during the later days of the British raj The Writers' was made the secretariat of the Government of Bengal.

Three young Bengali revolutionaries, Benoy Basu, Badal Gupta and Dinesh Gupta, entered The Writers' Building on December 8, 1930 and shot Col Simpson dead. Simpson was a notorious Inspector General of Prison. They were overpowered after a brief battle with the cops. Badal took potassium cyanide and died instantly. Benoy and Dinesh shot themselves. Benoy died after five days. Dinesh survived to be hanged later. The downtown of Calcutta, previously called Dalhousie Square, named after Lord Dalhousie, was rechristened as BBD Bagh.

I was not expecting a fancy office. In fact, he had an open office with many officers and clerks sitting with piles of files on their desk. He sat on a corner, indicating that he was a senior officer. I went to him with batted breath. I could hear the *dhak dhak* beats of my heart, pumping heavily. I gathered courage, folded my palm, as was the practice with us to show respect, and introduced myself. He was not surprised. He looked at me for a few seconds and signaled me to sit. His personality and command was obvious. He sat straight on his chair. A well-built body even then, must have been a very strong and impressive young man. Some of his colleagues were looking up with interest. Suddenly, the noisy environment became quiet. Many pairs of ears tuned to hear our conversation.

There was silence for some time. I attempted to start my rehearsed 'presentation' but looking at the face and kind of welcome expression on the face of this formidable personality, I waited. I gave him the option to start. He asked me about my parents and relatives, our residence in East Bengal and all that. I politely replied. I told him about my father's occupational history, about my family, which existed in the past, except my aunt and married sister at present. I told him about my ICSSR fellowship, the progress made in my research works. Told him about the vague plan about my future – that I would like to be involved in Economics research related work. I mentioned that I had applied for the position of Urban Economist in the Ministry of Planning & Development. I had also applied to a few other organizations. He listened intently. I had a feeling that perhaps he did not altogether dislike me. There was silence in between. We must have been thinking about the next topic for continuing the conversation.

Then abruptly he stood up and told me to come with him. I naturally followed. All necks from the surrounding tables craned to see us moving out. I thought he might be showing me the door. I followed him quietly. He might be thinking how to get rid of me in decent way. We landed in the large office canteen. He signaled me to sit opposite to him on an empty table. He called the waiter and whispered something. The waiter was respectful to him. A minute later, the waiter placed a plate with two pieces of mutton cutlets in front of me. He asked me whether I would have a cup of tea as well and ordered. I politely mentioned whether he would not have anything to eat. He had a slight smile and said not now. My heart was moving fast. However, my anxiety was almost gone. I finished my snack fast. The waiter came from nowhere with two cups of tea. Sipping his tea, he said, "I shall discuss with my wife and come back to you."

I could realize his mind must also have been moving fast. He must be thinking about his daughter's future with a person like me, who might be having a potential, which may or may not be achieved. That bright looking young man standing before him and asking for his daughter's hand was just one lone man in the world, with no material possession, not even a home!

My impression of him was great. The man wearing *kurta* and *dhoti*, a former astute freedom fighter, a brilliant student himself, who could have had a prosperous career, but sacrificed his youth and his career for fighting out the British government from our country. I left him standing there like a pleasant looking silent Buddha. In fact, he had won me over.

Tapati was waiting outside The Writers' Building with great concern and anxiety. How her father received me? Would he shout me out? He was fully capable of doing that of course. She asked all kinds of questions even without looking at me properly. I remained silent. My expression was easy, and relaxed with a sign of relief. After seeing me, she held my hand and asked, "Tell me what happened." I just said, "He treated me with mutton cutlet and tea!"

"Unbelievable!" She exclaimed. Hearing my detailed report, she felt both happy and anxious. Mother had to agree.

Meanwhile, I got a call for interview from West Bengal Public Service Commission for the position of Urban Economist. The interview went on for a long time of over 45 minutes, very unusual for such a position. The Chairman of the Commission was a very reputed person. He asked me many questions. My Narendrapur background was explored at length. Sometimes, there were arguments with the Chairman of the Commission. I did some plain speaking in reply to some of his provocative observations. I replied in a firm and straightforward way, albeit in a soft tone. I was not diplomatic in narrating my points of view. When it was over, I thought the game was gone.

To my sweet surprise, a message came from Bada Maharaj. He received an informal communication from somewhere (source not revealed) that the commission selected "a bright student from Narendrapur". I was thrilled. I told Tapati, who in turn informed her parents.

Bhabaranjan uncle and Shanti auntie visited Tapati's parents. My uncle was also a freedom fighter belonging to the *Jugantar* Group. Shanti auntie was also involved in the freedom struggle. I was staying with them for a few months when my Dover lane mess was shut down. They established a warm comradely relationship with Tapati's parents.

I decided to move from my uncle's place. I looked for a rented flat. It was difficult for a bachelor to get a rented flat. Eventually, I got one flat in a building called Pushpa Kuthi, Garia, owned by one of my uncles' friends. The flat was on the fourth floor and very airy; it was open on three sides. We could see the vast track of field up to the horizon lined up with green trees. In fact, we already knew Garia because of our Narendrapur connection. The house was located on the West side of the Tolly's Nala. It was a stagnant pool of dirty water across the Nala, a sort of a canal. I moved from my uncle's place to Pushpa Kuthi, sometime in the mid November 1973.

Historically, the course of the river Ganga used to flow from this canal. Shri Chaitanya Mahaprabhu (1486–1533), a great spiritual leader over 500 hundreds years ago in Bengal, spread Vaishnavisim, a version of Hinduism where members of all communities could worship, pray, and become a devotee of Lord Krishna. He used to sing "*Hare Rama, Hare Krishna*" with his devotees and dance, and travel across the country. A.C. Bhaktivedanta Swami Prabhupad founded the present 'Hare Krishna' movement under the banner of the International Society of Krishna Consciousness (ISKON). He was a follower of Vaishnavisism. It was on record that Shri Chaitanya traveled by boat on this branch of Ganga. There is a place adjacent to Garia, Vaisnavaghata, in south Calcutta.

Mythologically, Chand Saudagar, the legendary Bengali merchant used to sail his boats, full with merchandises, to trade with Sri Lanka and beyond. The story of Manasa Mangal is a story of Chand Saudagar, who refused to worship the mythological deity Manasa, the goddess of snakes. Manasa took revenge by sending a poisonous snake through a skillfully made tiny hole on the ceiling and bit Chand's son Lakhsinder on his wedding night. Chand had built the house with all precaution. However, the architect kept a tiny hole at the instance of Manasa. Behula, as the legend says, took the dead body of Laksinder on a long journey through this very route of the then high flowing river Ganga, which is now Tolly's Nala, a breeding ground of mosquitoes. The journey was for getting back her husband's life. As it happens in mythology, eventually the deity wins. Chand Saudagar worshiped Manasa. Thanks to Behula's efforts, Lakhsinder got his life back.

There are several 'ghats', which have names from Manasa Mangal. I read that Behula broke her journey on these places, located on the banks of the river Ganga. I visited some of these areas along with a sociologist friend of mine, who had written books on the historical aspects of the Manasa Mangal mythology.

When I was in Dhubulia, I had to read out Manasa Mangal during the monsoon season, a couple of chapters a day. Neighbors would collect in the evening and I would read out rhythmically. It used to be common practice in East Bengal. The reading followed a Puja of the deity Manasa.

The orthodox belief was that if the snake Goddess was happy with one's worship, snakes would not bite. The practice also protected snakes. People would not usually harm a snake unless it was about to bite. Since a snake's favorite food was rat, the existence of both balanced the ecosystem.

I hired some furniture. There was no arrangement for cooking. I had an electric kettle, a gift from Iain, which helped me to make coffee. I managed my lunch out but the problem of dinner was solved, thanks to Nani da, an ex-student of Narendrapur and his wife. Nani da was a known football player. He worked in a public sector bank. It just happened that they stayed near my flat in Pushpa Kuthi. Nani da and

Bhabi cordially invited me for dinner. Good souls are there; they make the world livable.

My uncle and aunt decided to arrange the marriage ceremony at their place. It was gracious of them to insist on organizing my marriage in their house, a grand gesture that I do always remember. That was a great relief for me. Tapati's folks would know that I am not alone in the world.

On the wedding evening, I told my father-in-law that I had received the appointment letter for the job of Urban Economist, a 'Class One Gazetted Officer' as it used to be designated during the British days yet continued until the 1970s. It implied that such category of high officers would be entitled to draw their own salary from the exchequer. In that sense, it was a prestigious category of service. However, the kind of complex form that one had to fill for drawing one's salary or TA/DA, would take away all fun. I got to know that later. That practice also continued until the 1970s.

I felt that he was relieved. He told me briefly, "I know you will get it." The marriage ceremony was colorful. I invited some of my relatives and friends. Over 200 people turned up and the food was excellent. The wedding reception was held at my uncle's place. I invited 100 people, I could not afford more. My elderly aunt came from Dhubilia. My sister and her family also came. Dr. S.N. Sen, then Vice Chancellor of Calcutta University, graced the occasion with Mrs. Sen. My supervisor S.B. Mukherjee and his wife also came.

We moved to Pushpa Kuthi with Tapati along with my aunt, who had come from Dhubulia for attending our wedding. Tapati did not allow her to return. We set up a home with our small means, decided to manage our expenses with our combined income, which, of course, was not high.

I discussed with my supervisor about my taking up the new job. He congratulated me for the job. He said, "Beating several qualified and experienced internal candidates you are selected. I am proud of you."

He advised me to take up the job. He added that a class one gazetted officer's job might not be available even after I successfully completed my research project. The offer had come at the right time. It was a prestigious assignment, with a good designation. He also told me that this job of Urban Economist could be a launching pad for my next job, if I wish to move over.

I surrendered my ICSSR Fellowship as advised. Otherwise, I could not accept the job. Considerable amount of my research work was almost complete. I thought I would be able to do the remaining on my own.

Events turned out differently later. My supervisor left the country for an indefinite period. I was shocked and I needed to get a new supervisor. However, due to political unrest the Senate of Calcutta University did not meet for almost a couple of years. The change of PhD supervisor needed the approval of the Senate those days. By then the latest housing census data was released, making my work outdated. Meanwhile, my life and career started transitioning on a different trajectory.

Once my medical and police clearance was obtained, within a month's time I received the formal appointment letter from the Hon'ble Governor's office.

CHAPTER 22

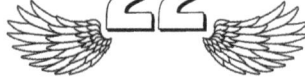

Planning for Santaldih Region

I sit erect, do some deep breathing and facial massage; try to organize my mind about things that happened to my personal life after I left Narendrapur. I think about the transition towards entering a career, try to take stock of the compulsions.

I had my first proper job and my father would have been happy if he were alive. I reached Asansol one day in the middle of February 1974 by early morning train from Howrah station. Asansol is the second largest city after Calcutta. It is a small city compared to the large metropolitan city, Calcutta. Asansol is 200 kms away from Howrah. It had population of only 1.2 million compared to Greater Calcutta's over 14 million in 2011. Asansol has several industries like iron and steel, coal and cement. It is an important hub of railway transport. The name Asansol has been derived from *'Asan'* trees which are seen in plenty across Damodar river and *'Sol'* meaning mineral enhanced land.

Next morning I went to APO office in Evelyn Lodge, once a beautiful house with surrounding areas, opposite the office of the Coal India Ltd, on the right side of GT Road. I entered the office but there was nobody occupying the desk of the receptionist on the ground floor. I moved up to the first floor, it was virtually empty. My enthusiasm was dampened.

Eventually, walking past the passage I found Amitava Bhattacharyay, executive engineer, in a corner of the office. He was a fair complexioned, medium height and elegant looking Bengali *Bhadralok* (gentleman). I introduced myself. He received me warmly. After the preliminaries, he took walked me across the office. He took me around and introduced me to few persons present.

I could not join service that day because the head clerk, who was in charge of keeping the 'joining form' in his custody was absent. It was a formality that I must sign the joining form before entering the government service. Amitava told me that the director, APO's administrative head, an IAS officer, N.B. Basak visited the office one day in a week. He actually was the full time director of Durgapur Development Authority. He came from Durgapur on the scheduled day of the week to APO, travelling by car a distance of 44 kms each way.

After waiting two days, I could join the office. The director was also there. We had a long conversation. He was happy to see another person joining APO. He told me frankly that during recent years no major work was being done in the APO. He was hopeful that probably a major project would receive approval from West Bengal State Electricity Board. He was a part time director, mandated to visit the office only one day every week, largely for signing some official papers. He was aware that office atmosphere was chaotic.

I interacted with other officers and staff members of about 20 persons in the socio-economic research division, which I would head. The APO also had an engineering division, a survey division and admin staff, in all over 100 people. Amitava introduced me to Ranjan Bhattacharyay, regional planner and Nakul Sadhukhan, assistant engineer. Both of them joined some months before me. They were very warm and friendly persons.

We also had Swadesh Chakraborty, a senior engineer – a nice person and older than us. Besides, there was one research officer in the socio-economic division, Shakti Gorai, an old timer. Four young research assistants recently joined my division as junior research assistants. In fact, some more people were also recruited in various categories in the recent months, which were popularly known as 'political recruitments', meaning that they had political patronage of the ruling Congress party.

I was in good company. The APO is a town and regional planning organization. Therefore, the technical officers must be very qualified persons. During my stay, I had an opportunity to meet and interact with a large number of engineers and several other technical officers in Asansol, Purulia and the adjacent areas where there was coal mine, coal washeries, power plant and related industries. Many of them were very hard working and committed persons.

In the weekend, I went back home. Tapati was waiting for me. The separation for the five days in a week was difficult to bear for both of us. We had just set up our first modest home. She worked as cartographer with NATMO. The job helped her to gain professional grounding, which helped her immensely in the future.

During that time, there was a month long railway strike all over India under the leadership of George Fernandez. As result, my weekend journey became hellish. I had to take a private bus or some other odd transport for travelling from Asansol to Calcutta on Saturday afternoon and back to Asansol on Monday morning. That was a distance of over 200 kms one-way by road, taking over six hours. I had to travel through the historic Grand Trunk Road, starting in Bangladesh, stretching across East, North and West India, then moving through Pakistan, and eventually ending in Kabul, Afghanistan. It totally covered a distance of 2,500 kms. It is now National High Way 2.

We read in history that the Grand Trunk (GT) was originally constructed during the Maurya Empire; third century B.C. Sher Shah Suri (1486–1556), founder of the Suri Empire in north India, took the initiative to reconstruct it almost as new road in the 16th Century. Thereafter, Lord William Bentinck had done it up during 1833–1860, giving it the present shape. Though Rudyard Kipling magnanimously praised this great road, as "… Such a river of life as nowhere else exists in the world", I could not enjoy my journey by GT Road. It was too narrow and clogged with traffic.

My mind was at home. We made a home! Tapati was alone with my old aunt. Often she would wait for hours for me at Garia bus stop in the evening. When the rail strike started, it was uncertain when I would reach. One night I reached Esplanade, Calcutta's down town area, at 1 am. I had to change four transports. There was no transport available to go to Garia. I saw a police van, approached and showed the police officer my government Identity Card. He carefully studied my ID, looked at my face and asked why I was so late. After hearing my ordeal, he helped me to reach home. Cops in Calcutta were very helpful in those days. I saw that the light was on the third floor of Pushpa Kuthi. Tapati was sweetly surprised. My aunt was also awake.

After spending a few weeks in the office, I became depressed. It was a moribund organization. I was told that letters were written to a number of sister organizations two months ago offering our services as a planning unit. Only one reply arrived and that was from the Chairman of West Bengal State Electricity Board. It was our good luck that he assigned us the big task of preparing a master plan for the Santaldih Region of Purulia district. Incidentally, the Chairman mentioned appreciatively that in his long civil service career, he had not received such a letter! I was thrilled that I would be very closely involved in that work.

A master plan for Santaldih meant that we would have to prepare a long-term perspective plan, or a comprehensive spatial plan for the sustainable development of the region. A master plan, according to some experts, provided a structured vision for the future for the region and the community. It also recommended appropriate land use plan for various activities, like different types of agriculture, industry along with its numerous categories, business, commerce, sports and recreation, residence as well as green zones. The ultimate objective of preparing a master plan for the region was to ensure welfare of the people and its encompassing habitat. In our case, we would have to prepare a master plan for the Santaldih of Purulia district.

Purulia district had a long heritage. The Jain *Bhagwat Sutra* in the 5th century mentioned Purulia as one of the 16 *Mahajanapadas*, a part of *Vajrabhumi*. It was part of Manbhum area comprising of Bankura and Bardhaman, a large area, during the early part of the British rule. Largely speaking, Manbhum district is what Purulia is at present. To cut a long story short, after India's Independence, Purulia district became West Bengal in 1956. It is the Western most district of West Bengal. With its tropical location, during summer temperature rises very high, sometimes above 50 degree Celsius. About 50% of the rainfall flows away as runoff. The district is 'covered mostly by residual soil formed by weathering of bed rock'.[1]

The population of Purulia was 2.9 million in 2011 census, with a density of 470 per sq kms, less than half of West Bengal's very high density of 1,028 sq kms. Because of the unwelcome weather and land conditions, Purulia lacked in agriculture. Major allied agricultural sector were silk and lac, and produces thereof. There were several industries in certain areas of Purulia namely, sponge iron, steel, cement and power plants. Tourism was also a great attraction. There were several rivers and rivulets like Kangsabati, Subarnarekha and the mighty Damodar. There were many lakes and small dams, and hills like the Ajodhya Hills.

During the spring season, Purulia became gorgeously beautiful with fully blossomed *palash, kusum and mahul,* all orange-red flowers of fire. It was a wonderful experience to see those bright flowers on the branches of trees and a red carpet created by those that fell on the ground, and, over and above, the setting sun making the sky glow in various shades of red. It was Nature's celebration – the festival of red!

What made Purulia famous were its *Chhau* and *Jhumur* dances and songs. *Chhau* dances are Indian tribal martial dances based on the themes taken from our great epics Ramayana and the Mahabharata. Participants dance wearing gorgeously colorful and huge masks as well dresses. *Chhau* dances are of three styles namely, Seraikala, Purulia and Myurbhang in Odisha. It has been inscribed in the UNESCO's 'Representative list of Intangible Cultural Heritage of Humanity'. *Chhau* dances are also an important cultural event of Odisha and Jharkhand.

Jhumur dances and songs also are yet another manifestation of Purulia and adjacent districts and states. Colorfully dressed young tribal girls hold their hands, form a semi-circle and dance to the tune of *Jhumur* songs, accompanied by male folks playing the drums and flutes. The lyrics of Jhumur songs are based on daily life and local themes sung in the local language.[2]

Santaldih Thermal Power Plant with installed capacity of 4x120 MW, of which, one unit was commissioned on January I, 1974 i.e., at the time we were doing our master plan project. Three other units were commissioned by 1987. Unfortunately, all four units were found to be 'non-functional' and were demolished! Subsequently, 6 and 7 units were commissioned.

Santaldih area was located amidst coalmines, coal washeries and certain other related industries. The small Santaldih township had an area of 350 acres, the power plant 800 acres and the ash pond 100 acres. People working there had a difficult time, particularly those living with families.

It was planned that four units of thermal power plant would generate electricity for the state. The power sector would play the role of a catalyst for the economic growth and development of not only Santaldih Township but also a Purulia district. The idea was great but as was seen later, the implementation was not.

For us there were some problems in our office for doing the master plan project. The first, hurdle was the initial reluctance of people in the office for doing the work. For seven years no substantive project work was done. It was not easy to make employees agree to work.

The socio-economic research unit members gave me a polite representation. Their union leader, also a member of the administrative staff, Amit babu (not real name), headed the representation. He stood in front my office with others behind him. He politely refused to take a seat and told me in a very friendly tone that they had heard that we were taking initiatives to do some major project work. Throughout his talk he frequently used 'Sirs' – perhaps deliberately. His mannerism still rings in my ears.

Amit babu replied to all my points in a very nice and sober but firm way. I told them nicely but firmly, "I'm fully aware what you just said, yes, I cannot do anything at all even if you do not work under the given circumstances. I am new here. There are four new young persons, who have recently joined as research assistants. Some of them are my juniors from the Department of Economics. I'm sure you will not stop them, if they agree to work with me."

He haltingly said, "Well, fine, perhaps, they can, if they wish." I realized that he was not ready for this. Four young faces were restlessly walking around. I could see them from my office. They must have heard Amit babu. They had a smile on their relieved faces. In fact, they were junior students from the Departments of Economics from both Jadavpur and Calcutta Universities.

The representation was over. I changed the topic and tone of conversation. I requested Amit babu to take a seat. I thought I should establish a rapport with him as he was a leader. He came in, sat and waived others to leave. I asked him about the office work in the past. I heard that some good projects were done at APO.

Amit babu sipped his cup of tea and went back to the past. He told me that there were several senior officers as Urban Economist, Regional Planners and Transport Planners. They left within a couple of years. I came to know later that CMPO/ APO was sort of launch pad for many of those young specialists. They came to APO for their grounding and left to other parts of India with a better job profile. In the past, some good projects were done in APO for the development of Asansol including a truck terminal. Then he said smilingly, "Sir, you will also not be here for a long period of time; if I may say so." He became emotional and added, "Sir, when we were young, we too thought that we would work for the country." He spoke at length and was almost in tears. At the end, he wished us good luck. We became friends. We, meaning Amitava, Ranjan and I. We started preliminary planning and had to go to Purulia, the district town frequently. It was a distance of about 85 kms by State Highway 5 via Raghunathpur. The distance from Purulia to Santaldih was about 43 kms. If we had to go to Santaldih directly from Asansol, it was a distance of 71 kms via Purulia Road through Raghunathpur Road.

We had to travel all these destinations several times to meet concerned experts and talking to people living there. Eventually, we prepared a questionnaire based on socio-economic as well technical survey work. It was an experience of a lifetime. All four of us got very seriously involved in the project.

We also had to the visit CMPO office and the office of the State Planning Board to consult experts. I came to know that the Ministry of Planning and Development had no legislative mandate for ensuring its plans were implemented. Each ministry like the Ministry of Industry, Agriculture and PWD had their own planning cells. They prepared their respective cost effective plans within the district.

For example, if the PWD department of Purulia district planned to build a road, it would take the shortest route. However, if the road was to be connected with the adjacent district/s, the length might have to be increased or the route changed. The concept of regional planning needed to take care of a larger area rather than keeping it restricted to just one district, but the district authority would have to take a cost effective approach. That was a systemic rigidity.

A regional plan had to take care of the future growth as well as the growth potential of the adjacent regions. For example, when we do a regional plan for Santaldih area, we should take care of the adjacent regions also. In the absence of the legislative mandate, the plan documents prepared by our Ministry were discussed in seminars, lauded by many experts and eventually shelved, at best they were taught at the academia abroad.

That was an important lesson for our team. We discussed the issue among ourselves. We decided to integrate plans made by specific Ministry offices in Purulia district such as Industry, Agriculture and PWD within our overall plan.

In our system, if the cabinet approved Santaldih master plan, a Santaldih Development Authority would have to be created for its implementation. At that time, the prepared plan might naturally have to be revised and changed to take care of real life issues. It was a long journey for the implementation of any such plan that we were preparing.

While Amitava and Ranjan were concentrating on engineering and structural aspects, I was involved with the socio-economic issues. I took great pain to sit with the heads of the concerned Ministry offices in Purulia. I realized that those people had intricate knowledge and understanding about their assigned areas of responsibilities. I discussed with each one of them for long hours on several rounds to learn, absorb details so that my components of the master plan would be realistic and implementable, at least by the respective segments like Industry, Agriculture or PWD as already mentioned. Our job was to attempt to integrate the relevant components of plans of various districts into our master plan.

Based on all that my specific recommendations would follow. We discussed with some experts in the State Planning Board. There were experts of various types. For example, there was an agriculture expert, Pannalal Dasgupta, who would give emphasis only on agriculture. For him even uttering the word 'industry' would result in a verbal onslaught. I had to face his onslaught on couple of occasions. We did not argue with him. It would be pointless. He was really an expert in his field, agriculture and rural development. I carefully took note of his points. We surely would ignore his biases.

Along with that, we received very pertinent inputs and advices from Prof. A.N. Bose, yet another member of the State Planning Board. He was earlier teaching at IIT Khargpur. Similarly, we discussed with many experts including my research guide, S.B. Mukherjee, who had wide understanding about regional planning issues. In fact, we invited him to come to our office and discuss with us. He came over for two days and we had lively discussions. His suggestions were very helpful in preparing our project.

I tried my best to sieve out the essences of those suggestions for the purpose of objectivity to incorporate in our plan proposals.

While I got deeply involved in my office work, I intend to mention that my living in Asansol was not easy. I had to stay five working days of the week and used to go home on weekends. I could not get any small flat on rent. Indian Iron and Steel Company (IISCO) occupied all vacant flats for their staff after its recent nationalization. I had to move from one duck bungalow to another including the guesthouse of Coal India. Eventually, I moved on to the terrace of Green Hotel near Asansol station, right on GT Road. There were half a dozen tiny, dwelling units on the terrace, with very low ceiling; available on rent. In the summer, it used to be very hot in Asansol, with temperatures rising up beyond 40 degree Celsius. Food was bad, very bad, and the stay was uncomfortable. Tapati visited for a few days. I took her to nearby areas including the DVC. A visit to the banks of Subarnarekha River was interesting. She was shocked to see my accommodation. We went back to the Coal India guesthouse for a few nights.

Life in Asansol had some disturbing dimensions. One was that if you kept your flat/ house open, everything would be stolen. However, reliable guards were available to guard your house. If those guards were not hired, then there was a risk of your house getting broken.

During the month I joined APO, the government recruited some employees in categories of class three and four as so-called 'political' candidates, i.e. those who served the ruling party before it occupied office. One of them was as an office 'peon'. He only had a right arm as he had lost his left arm in an 'accident' – people rumored street fight. People told me in whispers that he was a notorious person.

The point of concern for me was that he was assigned to me as my office peon. Chakraborty da and many others advised me not to ask him even for a glass of water.

The one-armed peon Brajen came to my office one morning. He apologetically requested me to get up from my chair. He cleaned the table, chair, the shelf, the floor – all with one hand. He positioned the chair and requested me to take my seat. He fetched a glass of water. I noticed the glass was dry. I realized that he knew how to serve water and thanked him.

He used to come in the morning to attend to my small amount of work. I knew he would disappear after sometime. One day he said that if I took a flat, I should inform him. He would see to that nothing went wrong in my flat even in my absence. My colleagues were surprised seeing Brajen working for me, talking to me in a friendly tone. They warned me that there must be some plan and asked me to be careful. I thought that there was nothing to be worried.

For two consecutive days, Brajen was absent. I heard that there was a fight between two rival groups and Brajen received serious injuries. He was in hospital. Chakraborty da told me not to be concerned about it. Such incidents did happen. Nevertheless, in the evening I told our driver to take me to hospital. Driver Dasarath was a nice person as well a smart driver. Dasarath looked at me and asked, "Sir, are you serious?" I smiled and repeated.

On reaching the hospital, I saw Brajen in the bed with lots of bandages on several parts of his body. A few of his relatives were also there. Brajen was conscious. He was so surprised that he wanted to get up, but I stopped him. His wife touched my feet. I asked them if I could do anything. They did not answer. I told him and his wife whatever was appropriate for such occasions. I gave some money to Brajen's wife for taking care of expenses.

That was big news in the office the following week. A recovered Brajen returned to office, profusely thanked me and touched my feet in presence of many people. He remained loyal and faithful to me. Chakraborty da came to my office and told me that I had done something unbelievable.

Amitava, Ranjan and I decided to go to Purulia town and Santaldih to clarify certain points. One was relating to our proposal for recommending a small dam on a rivulet. I also had to sit with the head of the Industry Department.

In Purulia, I arranged for our stay in the guesthouse of the reputed Ramakrishna Mission Vidyapeeth, Purulia, where our Parameshwer da was initially headmaster, and later, secretary. He received us with great warmth. We spoke a lot about our days in Narendrapur.

On our way to Purulia, almost half way through we saw an old potter crying on the road with his broken earthen pots. We stopped and spoke to him. He was carrying over a dozen earthen water containers on two sides of a bamboo stick supported on his shoulder. Each container was large enough to contain about 10 liters of water. He missed his step and fell down on the ground. He was going to the local *hat* (informal sector fortnightly market) to sell his merchandise. All his pots were broken. He was crying like a child. "These were my work of two weeks and I was planning to sell all my pots. There is huge demand for these pots, which keeps water cool in the summer season. But all are gone," he wailed.

We offered him some money. He refused, but we insisted. Eventually he took it thankfully and said, "Babu, we are very poor." His look, tearful face and words still do haunt me. For the three of us the poor potter was the symbol of poverty in rural Bengal.

My involvement in that assignment was so deep rooted that I used to have dreams at night. I saw in a dream that the Santaldih Development Authority (SDA) was formed and developmental activities were going on. I told my three close colleagues about it. They became speechless for some time. Ranjan said with a sad smile, "If wishes are horses, we shall have the SDA."

Yes, usually wishes are not horses. I know the difference between dream and reality. The dream reflected the desirable scenario. All dreams are not achieved in real life. So keeping the dream aside, I concentrated on the completion of my assigned job. The revised draft was ready. I asked my team, individually as well as group wise, to carefully go through the revised draft and prepare a list of further revisions, improvements and deletions. I also did the same. Then I consolidated the list of changes and inserted the corrections and changes. Those were the days of typewriters, internet, desktops and laptops were beyond even dreams. Within the next two weeks i.e., by the end of November 1974, my part of the master plan was ready.

Once my allocated portion of the assignment was completed, I left the document aside for a few days. Dr. Radha Kamal Mukherjee told me "…keep the pre-final version aside for some time and try not to think about it for a few days. Then sit with the papers and read it carefully all by yourself, think over what further improvement you would like to do, incorporate the changes and submit it."

During that period of gap, I took leave for a couple of days along with the weekend. I discussed with Tapati about changing my job. She was aware about the hassles of my job though I was really enjoying the present assignment. My accommodation and food in Asansol were miserable. So was the weekend travel. Besides, I knew another round of begging for an assignment would not work out.

Coincidentally, I came across an advertisement from Tata Services Ltd (TSL) in the '*Economic Times*'. They wanted to hire young economists for their Economics Think Tank. I decided to apply.

23

Prolonged De-Industrialization in West Bengal

'To most people sky is the limit. To those who love aviation, sky is home'
– Anonymous

The Bengali renaissance took place during the 19th and early 20th century. It was a unique reform movement encompassing religious and social reforms, art, culture, literature, science and patriotism. It was a great transition from the medieval to the modern. It did touch the area of commerce, business and industries as developed under the enterprising initiatives of 'Prince' Dwarakanath Tagore (1794–1846). Dwarakanath was one of the first Bengali industrialists and entrepreneurs, who started his business enterprises in as diverse areas as banking, insurance, shipping, coal mining, jute mills, tea plantation, indigo, urban real estate and *zamindari* estates largely in partnership with the British. He managed his large *zamindari* estate as a commercial enterprise, at times appointing British officers. He also set up a managing agency company. He was trading with the British, Parsi and Chinese. He was a 'Partner in the Empire' by his own right. However, "the business recession of the early 1840s and his newly acquired princely lifestyle led to the collapse of his business empire and made him a debtor".

Thus, what could have been a Tagore Group of companies in Bengal – like the formidable conglomerate, Tata Group, founded by Jamsetji Nusserwanji Tata (1839–1904) in 1868 in the Bombay Presidency – did not happen. Unfortunately, an Industrial Renaissance bypassed Bengal.

Prior to India's Independence, however, West Bengal was the top industrial nerve center of India, with large number of British and other corporate headquarters. Marwari businessmen were already there for about three centuries. Marwari moneylenders like Jagat Sheth used to lend money even to the Nawabs of Bengal.

Both large and small-scale industrial units were located in and around Calcutta, including Howrah, on the other side of the Hooghly river, popularly called Ganga. Howrah was the Sheffield of Bengal. Since Calcutta was the capital of British India until 1911, it also became the business capital of India. The industrial grandeur of West Bengal continued until the mid 1960s. A large number of people used to work in those industrial enterprises directly as well as indirectly in enterprises belonging to both forward and backward linkages of those industries. It generated income to a large number of employees, vendors and suppliers of all kinds, people involved across value chains of those numerous industries directly and indirectly. It generated huge resources and opportunities for many. That was a well-known story of the relative prosperity of Bengal before partition and West Bengal thereafter. It was the story of Bengal as the top industrial state in India.

That was also the story of one of the first overseas beneficiary of the second phase of the Industrial Revolution in England, which arrived here by default. For example, railways (1853), electricity (1897–1898), over land telegraph line (1850) and the British rulers introduced submarine cabling from Calcutta/Bombay to London (1870) in two decades of their commercial enterprise in India.

Of course, the primary objective for the introduction of those new technological innovations was to rule the vast country with an iron grip. As Benjamin Disraeli (1804–1881), twice Prime Minister of Great Britain, once stated: "…the British rule was not maintained for the benefit of the Indian nor simply for the sake of direct British interest in India; the Raj was there to keep firm the foundation on which much of the structure of formal and informal empire rested… the Indian empire should pay for itself and that Indian resources would be available in the imperial cause…"

That was it. Perhaps by default, it helped India to move over to the emerging new world.

Prior to India's Independence, Bengal was the top industrial state in India, close to Bombay Presidency (Maharashtra and Gujarat combined). In factory employment, West Bengal was at par with the Bombay Presidency during the 1940s. Calcutta was the head office of a large number of British, European and other multinational companies, including banks.

By the mid 1960s, West Bengal was second most industrialized state in terms of value-addition; it continued to remain on the top in factory employment.

After Independence, new the industrial investment moved to the Western and Southern states. Its share of net industrial value-added reduced to 14% in 1971 and further fell down to just 4% in 2002. The North-Eastern states including West Bengal became losers. For example, during the period of 1991 to 2003 the share of Gujarat in new industrial investment in medium and large-scale industries was as high as 16%, ranking second after Maharashtra, while the share of West Bengal was only 4%.[1]

Data from official sources on implemented investment indicate that during the 16-year period from 1992 through 2008, Gujarat ranked number 1 with Rs. 79.4 billion, followed by Maharashtra at a long distance (rank 2, Rs. 33 billion) and West Bengal (Rank 3, Rs. 30 billion).[2]

The investment situation changed by 2015 as states like Chhattisgarh, Andhra Pradesh and Karnataka moved up. Industrial investment intentions data show that Gujarat ranked 1st with Rs. 64.7 billion, a share of almost 21%, Maharashtra ranked 3rd with Rs 33.3 billion, a share of almost 11% and West Bengal had fallen to the 8th rank with Rs 17.7 billion, a share of just 5.7%. By 2016 Gujarat was 2nd with Rs 56.2 billion, a share of 13%, Maharashtra ranked 3rd with Rs 38 billion, a share of 9.3% and West Bengal fallen further to 9th rank with Rs 52 billion, a share of 1.3%.[3]

During the post Independent India the overall rate of growth of the state economy in general and industrial growth and development in particular suffered from the uneven rate of growth; different regions of India were growing at an uneven rate. This is despite ours having a centrally planned economy. West Bengal's planning model was revenue allocative model in nature, even though the availability of resources was left to 'desirable' estimates. The concept of 'space', which was important for the implementation of project, was unfortunately absent.

However, during the mid 1950s, i.e. after the First Five Year Plan (1951–56), there was some public investment in Durgapur, West Bengal, which "stimulated some growth but this was not enough to compensate for sluggishness of private investment", as pointed out by West Bengal Development Report prepared by the Institute of Development Studies, Calcutta for the Planning Commission.

Dr. B.C. Roy as Chief Minister took the initiative for the new industrialization of Bengal after Independence. Three public sector units, including Durgapur Steel Plant, an integrated steel plant, were established in 1955. An Alloy Steel Plant was established in 1965. Both the plants belonged to the Steel Authority of India Ltd. Besides, the Central Mechanical Engineering Research Institute and four powers plants including the well-known Damador Valley Corporation (DVC) were set up.

Pandit Nehru came for the inauguration and DVC officials selected two Santal girls to welcome Nehru. One of them, Budhni Mejhan, garlanded Nehru. He invited Budhni to press the button, the gates of DVC's Panchet Dam opened and water came gushing out. That naturally created big news in next day's newspapers. Unfortunately, Budhni was ostracized by her community. The community traditionally believed that a girl garlanding a man meant she was married to him. Besides, there was not a single member of their community at the inauguration. She had just one moment of publicity in history and later DVC sacked her! Subsiquently, a Bengali gentleman, Sudhir Dutta, married her. She approached Rajiv Gandhi in 1984 when he was Prime Minister. With Rajiv Gandhi's intervention, she got back her job.

Several other chemical and metallurgy plants were also started along with a CSIR lab and a reputed engineering college.

Durgapur is the second planned city in India, and the third largest city in West Bengal. Joseph Allen Stein and Benjamin Polk did the planning. Dr. B.C. Roy dreamed of the industrial city, which along with Asansol would be the second most important twin cities for industrialization of Bengal after Independence. Since many British industrialists had left India after Independence, the industrial growth and development started suffering. Under the circumstances, Dr. Roy took initiative to make Durgapur-Asansol a new industrial corridor.

In fact, under the auspices of Development and Planning Ministry, West Bengal Government, the CMPO was set up in 1961 to prepare a comprehensive development plan for the metropolis of Calcutta. The CMPO was the first of its kind in India. It prepared the famous Basic Development Plan of Calcutta for the 20-year period from 1966 to 1986.

Subsequently, APO and SPO were also set up in line with, and attached to, the CMPO. The Durgapur Development Authority was also set up for implementing the urban regional development plan proposals.

Over a period, there was a modest increase in the population largely due to migration from the catchment areas, adding developmental impetus through the natural route. The population of Durgapur was about 0.6 million in 2011 census, up from about 0.5 million in 2001. There were a number of engineering colleges, small and medium sized industrial units and shopping malls. Whatsoever growth and development happened in Durgapur was due largely to increasing demands of the changing time led by circumstances, and not because of any focused planned approach. In fact, the vision of making Durgapur a growing industrial hub did not materialize

Since the mid 1960s, the socio-political and economic situation in West Bengal became disturbing for a prolonged period, almost half a century. It is yet to come out from this impasse. The lengthy process of deindustrialization has taken such a nightmarish spell that it is difficult to predict when West Bengal would be able to wake up and see the light of the day.

Many of these industrial units were already old and were showing signs of wear and tear. Besides, the pressure of increasing population steadily arriving from East Bengal like a continuous flow of water created unimaginable problems. Political, social and economic situation in West Bengal became very chaotic and unmanageable. The rate of urban unemployment rate is as high as 40%. This persistent unemployment, both the huge stock and annual additions, led to the growth of the ugly lumpen class, who joined political parties and destabilized social life. No wonder political violence and criminal activities are rampant in West Bengal.

Thus, the entire North-East region including West Bengal was denied investment opportunities for industrial development. Besides, there were many other restrictive policies with respect to Eastern states like West Bengal, which were used for denial of industrial projects. Dr. Ashok Mitra as Finance Minister of the United Front (UF) Government vociferously took up these discriminatory treatment of Eastern states like West Bengal with the Union Government. The Union Government did not care to listen.

The ideological consideration of the Left parties discouraged the growth of industrialization per say mainly because of their labor-focused approach. As already discussed, the complex problem of economic rehabilitation of the refugees was not managed properly. Unrest among refugees went on increasing. Opposition parties took grievances of the refugees, organized agitations and movements against the Government on a regular basis. The need for more employment generation through setting up new industries was not on the agenda. Strikes, *bandhs, hartals, dharnas, gheraos*, tools & pen down and work to rule organized by militant trade unions were the order of the day. Violence at factory gates, inside factories, beating up company managers, throwing of hand bombs and taking 'care' of rivals and informers were rampant during that period. In a large company, there could be more than a dozen of unions. All that was done in the name of workers' right. Perhaps, that was expropriation of the so-called expropriators!

It was true that the management of certain companies nurtured a culture of exploiting workers, not paying them their due wages and bonus and harassing the workers in so many ways. Workers would come to work in the morning and see that the factory gate would be locked.

They would see a brief and cryptic notice pasted on the wall saying that the factory would remain closed for an indefinite period. Besides the recognized union, rival unions were created with the blessing of the management. 'Tension' was often infused among unions so much so that they were always engaged in fighting. There was always a cause and effect dilemma between the management decision and the union action/ reaction, and vice versa! The trust between the union and the management completely broke down.

This has been continuing over six decades, in West Bengal, from the mid-1960 until today, 2017, and would definitely continue in the near future.

Of course, there were a few small positives in between. Like the setting up of Haldia Petrochemicals Ltd, a joint venture with, the Government of West Bengal, the Chatterjee group, Tata Group and Indian Oil Corporation. It was approved in 1984; but was founded in 1994. Over a period, several other plants were setup. South Asian Petrochemicals, IOC, Exide, Shaw Wallace, Tata Chemicals and Mitsubishi Chemicals had already been set up.

Haldia Township, about 12 kms south-west of Calcutta, had some modest growth, with a small population of over 200,000 in 2011. The original objective was to set up a bulk cargo handling green port. Interestingly, the only mini Japanese township, Staku, was set up in Haldia. Under normal circumstances, Haldia by now should have been a considerably large industrial cum port township. That did not happen.

During the second half of the Left front Government's rule, some positive initiatives for setting up industries were taken. The West Bengal Government established the new Industrial Policy of West Bengal in 1993 for industrial development, rehabilitation of sick units, generation of employment and protection of legitimate interest of labor. The West Bengal Industrial Development Corporation (WBIDC) was set up as a single window to help new industrial investment in West Bengal. However, nothing materialized except signing of a number of Memorandums of Understanding with WBIDC.

First, the main Left party, CPI (M) leaders realized the importance of industries much late. During the first 25 years, they behaved in an unfriendly manner towards the cause of industrialization. They were happy with their focus on agriculture in general and land reform in particular. They looked at industry as their enemy. They solidly sided with the party affiliated trade unions.

Second, non – existence of a comprehensive land use policy; unless a proper land use planning/ mapping is done, land acquisition particularly for industrialization would be done at random or based on myopic administrative or political decisions. For example, multi-crop land should not be given to build industries, destroying generations old livelihood of farmers unless there was a pronounced better alternative. In this context, the stories of Nandigram and Singur are well known.

Jyoti Basu, Chief Minister for 23 years (June 1977 to Nov 2000), the legendary figure, understood the importance of industries rather late. He went abroad and other states of the country seeking industrial investment. In his ministry, there was Bidyut Ghosh, Industry Minister, who took some initiatives in this regard.

I personally remember that there was a meeting organized by Bombay Chamber of Commerce and Industry where Bidyut Ghosh spoke eloquently and invited industrialists present in the meeting to invest in West Bengal. Many industrialists, both domestic and foreign, attended the meeting. The hall was to full capacity. The Industry summit organized by Confederation of Indian Industries was held in Calcutta. There also many industrialists expressed their interest to invest in Bengal. But, the expressed intent was not implemented.

Then it was the turn of Buddhadev Bhattacharyay, Chief Minister for 11 years from 2000. His also realized late that industrial development was required. His first initiative was Nandigram, Purba Medinipur (aka Midnapore), a fundamentally low-lying agricultural area. The choice of the site was definitely wrong. The plan was to 'forcibly' acquire 10,000 acres of land based on the ancient land acquisition act of 1894 for setting up a SEZ to be developed by a little known Salim Group from Indonesia. Villagers resisted the forcible land acquisition, 14 villagers were killed and over 70 wounded by the police firing. One police officer was also killed and 14 other policemen were wounded. The project met a natural death.

Singur was yet another such tragic destiny. Tata Motors' small car Nano plant was to be set up in Singur, Hooghly district near Calcutta. Singur was also an agricultural land with multi cropping done in many plots. The State Government acquired 997 acres of farmland to give the acquired plot to Tata Motors. Though majority of landowners had already accepted the payment, some 400 plus people did not. Mamata Banerjee, leader of Trinamool, launched a strong agitation against the Tata Nano plant so much so that Tata Motor decided to shift the plant in 2008 to Sanand in Gujarat where the Government offered all help.

Eventually, the Trinamool Government came to power with a thumping majority under the leadership of Mamata Banerjee with one of the promises that the Singur land would be given back to farmers. She could hand over the land to farmers only in September 2016 after Supreme Court gave its verdict. Singur has now made an about turn from the prospect of becoming an industrially advanced region as against agriculture. The hands of the growth paradigm have moved anti-clockwise.

Economic growth and development of a densely populated state like West Bengal requires a comprehensive approach towards all three sectors – primary, secondary and tertiary. The approach should not be one or the other, or one against the other. Unfortunately, major political parties have missed this point. They have been playing a stubborn political game, playing favorite to one sector or the other – not that they loved one or the other; they only loved their perceived political interest.

It is relatively a small state with an area of 89,000 sq kms and a large population of 91.3 million, adding over 1.1 million persons per year! The State's agriculture is wide spread. It will be difficult to acquire huge chunks of land in a consolidated area for the purpose of large manufacturing industry without appropriate land use planning and mapping. The new Land Acquisition Act 2013 has made acquisition of land extremely difficult. The new 'realization' by the people in rural Bengal, inspired by Singur will make it difficult to acquire large areas of land for setting up industries.

During TMC rule, huge amounts of investment intentions were expressed at annual business summits organized by the State

Government. In the Bengal Global Business Summit of February 2018, investment intention of a huge amount of Rs. 2.8 trillion was talked about.[4] If talks and pledges were horses, Bengal would surely ride …

There are certain emerging realities, which are yet to be comprehended by the political and bureaucratic combine in the country as a whole and West Bengal in particular.

First, because of the imperatives of steep competition, the manufacturing sector has been improving productivities in all segments like labor, capital, input-output ratios and even total factor productivity (TFP), which has considerably increased. The TFP, as one may think, is not the combination of all other factors of productivities. It is, in fact, the measure of the contribution made by management and technology.

For example, 20 years ago in 1995–96, Tata Steel (operations in India) used to produce about 2.7 million tons of steel by employing over 72,282 employees. In 2015–16 Tata Steel's production in India increased by 3.6 times to 9.7 million tons of steel by employing only 35,439 employees, less than half of the number of employees in 1995–96. Thus, we needed 26,771 employees to produce one million tons of steel 20 years ago. Today, we need only 3,653 employees to produce one million ton of steel. That is to say, just one person could now do what 7.3 persons did 20 years ago… This is what labor productivity is. Similarly, all other productivity parameters have also improved significantly.

The point is that there is a productivity paradox here. Due to productivity increase, massive use of robots, increased automation and intelligent machines, the direct employment in manufacturing industry could not be increased. The objective is to increase per employee value addition, not increase the number of employees. If you watch the National Geographic videos on mega factories, you will not see rows of employees. You will see robots of all kinds, automated processes of manufacturing and only some employees in key areas. Thus, large-scale and direct employment generation is out of question in today's manufacturing industries. Of course, some direct employment will take place at the plant level, if investment takes place; there will be employment creation in the linkage sectors, both backward and forward, as well as in the small ancillary sectors.

In this context, it is also important that India's manufacturing competitiveness has not sufficiently grown, despite the Government's good intent. China became a global manufacturing hub for the developed world. The US manufacturing job has steadily declined from 17.6 million in 1990 to just 11.8 million in 2012. Perhaps, it is rather late to make 'Make in India' a grand success.

Second, digital – three dimensional – manufacturing activities have been replacing old style shop floors in a progressive way. This will radically change industrial operations in the immediate future.

Third, the historic growth model – the ascendency from agrarian growth leading to growth in manufacturing sector and then the growth of services sector – seems to have bypassed in case of India. This is true even in the case of West Bengal. The tertiary sector's contribution to West Bengal's GDP was as high as 58% in 2009–10. It is growing perhaps because it is the most apolitical and uninterrupted sector compared to the other two, agriculture and industry.

Fourth, in recent years the United States has lost more than 50% of its manufacturing operations to China for economic reasons of outsourcing production because of very low labor cost. This has caused huge job losses. And experts like Vaclav Smil think that further large-scale job loss can happen in the future in the USA due to automation and digital manufacturing.[5]

Our politician, bureaucrat and technocrat combine may carefully consider the new growth model for our immediate future. Where and how could we generate employment for millions of young people?

India's great demographic dividend of having the highest stock of young people (14 to 64 years age group) would require job creation for 869 million by 2020, according to an UNDP study. Over one million people are added to the work force every month! Inappropriate handling of this gigantic task would lead to endless chaos, unrest, violence and anarchy.

CHAPTER

24

Call from Mumbai

I had done right by resigning from Asansol Planning Organization as Urban Economist. If stayed on I would have rotted… Yet another announcement. Seat belt sign is on. The plane is facing an air pocket – you feel like a quick drop in the air, but rarely gain or lose more than 20 feet.

I received the interview letter in late November 1974. I was hoping the interview would be in Mumbai. I thought that I would be able to also explore certain others opportunities in Mumbai. But my interview would be held at the Tata Center, Calcutta.

D.R. Pendse, Economic Adviser (EA), Tata Services Ltd (TSL), conducted my interview. Two senior executives from Tata Group of companies also separately joined the process for some time. It went on for several hours, before and after lunch. So many topics were covered from economics, business, international affairs to politics and society that I was wondering where all those would lead to.

As advised, I went to Tata Center next morning. I was happy to hear that they had decided to recruit me as an economist in the Department of Economics and Statistics (DES), TSL in Bombay House, the corporate office of the Tata Group, in Mumbai. The appointment letter would reach me within a month. I quickly thought through the numbers. The starting salary of about Rs. 2,000 per month was fine in the mid 1970s. However, I would be staying in Mumbai and Tapati with my old aunt, at least for some time, would have to stay in Calcutta! Arithmetically, the doubling of salary would be neutralized by the doubling of expenses – for running two set ups.

Pendse briefly explained that the DES was the Think Tank of the Tata Group, set up by J.R.D. Tata, Chairman of the Tata Group companies, in the mid 1940s for helping corporate executives in analyzing and interpreting economic issues, forecasting the future, doing research projects in relevant and unexplored areas. He added that JRD was a visionary leader. He thought that India would be independent from the British rule. Industry, commerce and business would expand. The DES would play a supporting role towards this.

I came back home happy and worried at the same time. I told Tapati everything. Getting a better job was *sine qua non* (absolutely necessary). At the same time, the job was not in Calcutta, but in a far off place on the other corner of India, about 2,000 kms away. The fact was that we could like to move to Mumbai immediately. I had to first go alone, assess the job, its prospect, try to arrange a place to live and all that. Would money be enough to run two establishments? All such questions were racing up and down in our minds. Yet there was also relief in our minds that I had not failed in my endeavor. I had not failed Tapati and my father – in-law. I had not failed my father. I had not failed myself.

The next morning I went to Asansol. Except for one friend of mine, nobody knew about my interview. I told him that my interview was good. They would inform within a month either way. I concentrated on finishing and fine-tuning my part of the Santaldih master plan.

My part of the work involved the socio-economic aspects of the area, planning recommendations for industry, agriculture and services activities, making a detailed business plan, activity wise land use plan and forecasting future growth areas. I did that with my team and we spent long hours. By mid December 2004, our unit's part of the master plan was ready. However, I did not release it. Since I had the advantage of time on my side, I kept document with me to give a last look before submission.

I explained to the young research assistants certain tips of the game. For example, when doing a large-scale research project, first apply your mind to carefully understand the assignment details. Prepare the draft plan. Try to look for some published project reports and find out what and how they had been done. Taking lessons from those reports, you must do a better report in all aspects. Besides, you must finish the work before the deadline but do not submit it too soon. Use the time available for critically looking into the report and try to improve it.

The appointment letter arrived. I carefully went through the terms and conditions and the package of compensation. I had to accept it within three weeks.

Tearfully – because we would have to live separately for some time – we decided to accept the job. Another job of this kind would not be available as the economic and business situation in Calcutta was deteriorating fast. The overall economic condition in the country was also not at all encouraging. During the Fourth Plan period (1969–74), the real rate of growth of the economy was just 3.3%. Employment opportunities had virtually withered away. Industrial environment in West Bengal had deteriorated considerably and job opportunities dried up.

Even under such adverse business environment, I got another job as assistant secretary with a particular Chamber of Commerce, Calcutta. I learned from some senior students of the Economics Department, who worked with the Bengal Chamber of Commerce, the nature of the work in the Chamber of Commerce. They advised me to accept the chamber job only as a stopgap arrangement. I discussed with the secretary of the chamber, who was playing a mentor's role. With his good wishes, I decided not to accept it.

With tears in our eyes, Tapati and I decided to post the acceptance letter for the job offered by Tata Services. Initially, I would go to Bombay alone. Tapati had a job in Calcutta as a cartographer in NATMO, Government of India organization. She could not resign at that stage. Besides, my old aunt was there. Not all of us could go to Mumbai.

The following Monday I informed my colleagues at Asansol that I would submit my resignation letter after submitting my part of the master plan within a couple of weeks. They already knew that my portion of work was ready. There was quite an excitement about my leaving because my stay was the shortest as Urban Economist. I had not yet completed even one year.

Chakraborty da came to me separately and profusely wished me luck. He also told me that as per rules it would be easier to resign before the completion of one full year, as my service was not regularized yet – very sound advice.

I plunged into my part of the report and started carefully reading, revising and editing pages after pages for the final round. I, along with some of my juniors, formally submitted our part of the report to Amitava, executive engineer, our functional head.

When the director visited on the scheduled day of the week, I told him about the completion of my part of the Santaldih master plan. He was an IAS officer and our administrative head. As a student of Geology, he had his understanding about mineral resources of Purulia district. He leafed through the report and expressed his satisfaction about it. In fact, we were discussing contents of the report on many occasions. He was aware of the goings on.

Once the official formality about the report was over, I told him that I would like to submit my resignation soon. He was obviously shocked. "You are here for just about a year and would be leaving us," he asked.

"I am happy with this work. There will be no other work in the office once this report is submitted. The environment in the office without work will again be anarchic. Would you have continued if you were in my place," I replied.

He was silent for a few moments. Then he added, "It takes a long process and time to recruit an officer in a government organization. I was thinking about that."

I did not want to argue with him. I apologized for the inconvenience caused because of my sudden resignation and thanked him for his cooperation.

He smiled helplessly. Our conversation continued for some more time.

I told him briefly about my job with Tata Services. He listened carefully. Our conversation went on for quite some time. Finally, he wished me well on my new job.

Colleagues from my team and others bid goodbye; Amit babu bid goodbye and reminded me about his prediction. With so many people's good wishes, I left Asansol.

25

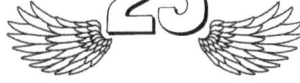

Joining Tata Services

This is Durga Puja time, the most gorgeous festival of Bengalis. Exquisitely made idols of the Goddess Durga, riding on a lion and posing to kill 'Mahishasur,' the demon, and accompanied with her four children, are worshipped with profound love and respect. Mythologically, the daughter and her children visit her parent's home.

Thousands of thematic as well as traditional pandols are made every year. They all look like magnificent pieces of art. Then after four days, the images are immersed and the pandols are broken down. We feel sad about the destruction of such gorgeous creative works. However, this is a continuity of art and culture in Bengal. Besides, Durga Puja generates huge economic activities for all kinds of people – artisans, idol makers, decorators and traders in Bengal. Literally, millions make money during this time for their whole year's living. Huge tourism potentials are there, but the problem is crowd – millions of people are out on the street – more so at night.

On February 14, 1975, I boarded the Howrah-Bombay Mail via Nagpur. Tapati, my father-in-law and some others were on the railway platform. Tapati's eyes were full of tears; so was mine. When the train rolled out of the platform, she ran with it as long as she could. I craned my neck back and kept on waving even after the train left the platform.

I reached Mumbai in the morning, Sunday, February 16, the day of Vasanta Panchami. The Bengali community performs Saraswati (Goddess of Learning) Puja on this day every year. Saraswati Puja is performed almost in every Hindu family, every educational institute and in the locality in Bengal. I have already mentioned about the Puja we organized in Dhubulia.

This was my second trip to Mumbai. When I came here in 1972, I hardly knew that Mumbai would be my home for life.

Ramen N. Ganguly, father of my ex-student Amit from Narendrapur, and Amit came to receive me at Dadar station. I had written to them about my job in Mumbai. They were very helpful. They had arranged my paying guest (PG) accommodation with the family of the late Tarun Bose, a popular character actor in Bollywood movies. Tarun's young son Arup was Amit's friend. They took me to Bandra West, a posh area, popularly known as the 'Queen of the Western' suburbs of Mumbai. Close to Almeida Park, there was a high-rise building, where on the seventh floor I got a fully furnished PG accommodation.

I came to know that film artistes and top technical persons do visit Arup's place. In later days, I had the opportunity to meet a number of them. Arup also told that the popular lyricist – of Hindi film songs – Anand Bakshi lived on the sixth floor just below theirs. Arup told me that around midnight probably his music system would be on; a pleasing wave of soft music would spread across some parts of the building. The lyricist would be engaged in composition.

The time of Saraswati Puja is very pleasant. The spring is transcending to winter season. Young girls wear lemon yellow colored saris, which perhaps is the first time for many of them. Boys are clad in white *dhotis* and *kurtas*. This also could be the time for some teenage boys and girls to meet and give shy dove-eyed looks at each other. It could be just the first time a boy 'likes' a girl or vice versa. It could be the beginning of their first love in some cases.

This is also the time for the initiation of handwriting for the kids. The kid usually sits on the lap of a priest in front of the deity. The priest helps the kid to scribble alphabets on a banana or palm leaf. This is the beginning of their schooling. Interestingly, they have some options to pick up – a pen, cash or gold ring. If the kid picks up a pen, it was believed that the kid would be attracted to studies; holding cash or gold ring would mean that the kid would go for riches.

Many devout Bengalis would offer *Anjali* – flower offering and prayer to the Goddess. The believers also fast before offering *Anjali*. After the *Anjali* was over, a special Bengali vegetarian food – *bhog prasad* or *khichari,* as it is called – would be served with *labra* (a Bengali dish made of mixed vegetables), *chutney* (sweet and sour) and *payesh* (a sweet dish made of rice).

Similarly, one week after Durga Puja – in the evening/night of *Kojagori (who is awake) Purnima (full moon)*, Lakshmi Puja is also performed almost in every Hindu Bengali family. It is worship of the Goddess of Wealth. Family members, particularly the mother of the house takes the lead role. Even today in many families, elderly women perform Lakshmi Puja every Thursday evening. They read aloud in a musical tune from a small booklet containing the prayer for the Puja. When I was young, I did that in our house in Dhubulia in the absence of my mother.

Amit took me to the Puja *pandol* of Vivekananda Club, Bandra, a club of the well-established Bengalis. On my first day in Mumbai itself, I came to know a large number of people from this gathering. Ramen Babu introduced me to many people.

I just stood there with a faint smile on my face, said a few words, but my mind was in Calcutta – thinking of Tapati. What was she doing on the day of Saraswati Puja? She might have gone to her father's place. She would get some company there.

Ramen babu introduced me to his friends. Some people also approached me and we exchanged pleasantries. Some young persons close to my age group were also there like Chaudhury, Shurhid, Manu and a few others. We decided to meet in the weekend and we soon became friends.

On my second morning in Mumbai, Monday, February 17, 1975, I formally dressed in a suit and a tie reported in Bombay House, the famous head office of Tata Group of companies to DES, TSL on the left side of the ground floor.

There was P.K. Sen, office superintendent, with whom I had spoken twice over telephone from Calcutta. I went to him and introduced myself. After the formalities, Sen took me to D.R. Pendse, EA – our boss, who sat in a closed cabin in one corner. He received me with warmth. We exchanged courtesies. He briefly explained about my work and said that he would discuss at length later.

Sen took me out and gave me a run down about the DES office, people working there and its history. He introduced me to everybody in the open office. There were three senior economists and four economists, one research assistant, one admin officer, one clerk and three secretaries. Along with four peons, the total strength working under the EA was 19 persons. I tallied the number with my previous office where more people were working under me.

I was led to a table and chair, my place to sit, at the end alongside two peons; one of them was cutting newspaper clippings, the other pasting them in classified files. I was shocked. I heard such glorious things about the Tatas from so many people that it became difficult for me to sit down on my allotted desk. It was the Writer's Building type of an office, only somewhat cleaner. The overall surrounding and the ambience were disappointing. Looking at how casually the male folks dressed themselves, wearing a suit and tie, I looked like the joker in the pack. Had I done the right thing accepting this job as against my previous job of a 'class one gazetted officer'?

Keeping my disturbing feeling bottled up, I quickly decided I would have to live with it, at least for some time. I went around and spoke to senior economists, those with large desks, as I had guessed. First, I went to V.S. Borwankar. Before joining DES, he worked with the Forward Market Commission where Pendse was his boss. Pendse brought him here. He specialized in industry and related areas. A soft-spoken person, he seemed helpful.

Then I met V.A. Shah, popularly called as Vinu Bhai or Shah Bhai, who specialized in public finance and stock market related matters. I understood that he was widely read and had an intellectual bent of mind. He was in the middle of reading of 'The Listener', the weekly BBC radio magazine. Alex told me about it. Seeing a copy in his hand, I told him that I had read a few copies but not regularly. He promptly asked the librarian Lata Rele to give me some copies. While conversing with him, he incidentally asked me whether I had read Gunnar Myrdal's 'Asian Drama'. I was sure he was testing me.

I told him that Myrdal was a formidable development economist, professor, sociologist and politician. He became minister of Swedish government number of times. He was also Executive Secretary, UNECSO. Three volumes of *'Asian Drama' – 'An Inquiry into Poverty of South Asian Countries'* – were landmark works of Myrdal. I told him about his getting the Economics Nobel prize in 1974 with Friedrich Hayek. A temperamentally 'socialist' Myrdal suggested the abolition of the Nobel Prize in Economics as some 'right reactionaries' like Hayek and Milton Friedman were awarded the prize. I guess I passed the test.

Lata, a smart and friendly person, gave me an idea about books, journals and government reports available in the library. She offered me some publications on the activities of the Tata Group companies to read. I needed them, as I did not have much idea about Tatas. I moved over and talked to all almost everyone in the office.

I left the office after 5 p.m. by the time most people had left. My mind was heavy and uncertain. I walked slowly across the Flora Fountain, rechristened as the Hutatma Chouk, the Martyrs' Square, symbolizing the death of 105 persons in police firing at the time of the Samyukta Maharashtra Movement in 1956 for the separation of the State of Maharashtra from the combined Maharashtra and Gujarat state of the Bombay Presidency. The movement was for the setting up of the Marathi speaking state, Maharashtra, which happened on May 1, 1960. Gujarat also became a separate state. My mind moved from the uncertain state to the historically important sites of Bombay's (now Mumbai) central business district (CBD).

Flora Fountain, the beautiful square in the middle of the CBD, was built in 1864. Flora was the Roman Goddess of Abundance, symbolizing Bombay's prosperity. The LIC building is on the meeting point of Mahatma Gandhi Road and Dadabhai Naoroji (DN) Road like the two forks of 'Y', facing the fountain.

Incidentally, Dadabhai Naoroji Road, in later years, was awarded the Heritage Road/Mile status. The road stretches from Crawford Market (wholesale market) to Victoria Terminus, now called Chhatrapati Shivaji Maharaj Terminus (CSTM), on the one side and the JJ School of Arts building and Greater Mumbai Municipal Corporation head office on the other. It finally reaches Flora Fountain. Many buildings on the road were constructed in the 19th century in 'Neo-Classical and Gothic Revival Style'.[(1)]

Moving southward from the Fountain, opposite the High Court of Mumbai building and HSBC bank is Homi Mody Road. The second building on the left of Homi Mody Road is the famous Bombay House, the seat of the corporate office of the Tata Group companies since 1924.

Bombay House was architectured by George Wittet, who designed 40 buildings for the Tata Group in various places in the city as well as elsewhere. George Wittet eventually joined to head Tata Engineering Company, now Tata Motors. This is the first heritage building, which has recently been awarded Green Rating as it conserved 35% of power since 2010. While thinking about all this, I also thought that I have joined an office located in this historic building. I just did not know then that I would work here for three decades in a row!

The other road from the Central Bank of India's office, opposite the High Court building leads to the old Bombay Stock Exchange building on Dalal (broker) Street, established on July 9, 1875. Presently, there is a 29-storey high rise building called Phiroze Jeejeebhoy Tower since 1980. The Fountain area is also called Fort, as there was a mile long wall built in 1769, called Fort George III, in the name of George III, the King of England. It was built for segregating white skinned people from natives.

I understood later that the new central business district is Nariman Point beyond the Churchgate station and Marine Drive. The land was made out after filling up ocean beds on the coastlines. Reclamation added to a huge acreage, ignoring the environmental consideration, which, of course, was not an issue then. I have seen the photograph of old Bombay, where the ocean was nearer to today's land mass of Azad Maidan.

The new CBD locates a large number of so-called modern high-rise buildings for both government and non-government offices. One of the landmark high rise – 23 storey – commercial towers was the Air India building. It was completed in 1974, just a few months before I came to Mumbai. With its red fluorescent logo of Air India, the Unicorn, the mythical winged horse – shines at night on top of this tall building located on Marine Drive at the edge of the Arabian Ocean. It was the head office of Air India until 2013.

Across Marine Drive, there are rows of low-height buildings, usually not more than four to five storeys with mixed land use. Commercial establishments were located on the ground floors and residential on the upper floors. A magnificent looking curve with shining lights seen from the Malabar Hills on the other end of the convex curve is called the Queen's Necklace! People walk on the tiled footpath, sit on the ramparts to cool their body and soul in the mild flowing evening breeze. You can look up to the sea line at the horizon.

The first ever departmental store in Bombay is also there. The Akbarallys at the Fountain area was originally set up in a small way in 1897 and subsequently expanded in 1956. Another such departmental store came up in 1976 opposite Churchgate station.

Talking about the convenience stores or organized retailing in India, I have my distinct memory that my Bhabaranjan uncle took us to the Kamalaya Stores, established in 1941 in Calcutta, where I enjoyed my life's first experience of eating in a fancy restaurant in 1948. I came to know later that the Spencer's introduced the first ever departmental store concept – their first store opened in Madras as early in 1863.

Walking across from Churchgate to Marine Drive, I saw one entrance gate to the Brabourne Stadium of the Cricket Club of India, built in 1937 where Test matches used to be played until 1972. The famous stadium with a seating capacity of 25,000, we heard in so many radio commentaries of Test matches, was in front of me! Subsequently, Wankhede stadium, with a capacity of 33,000, was built across Churchgate in 1974.

Being more of a football enthusiastic, I also saw the football ground at the Cooperage, with roofing over the main stand only and dilapidated wooden planks for the football loving public to seat. It was converted into a stadium in 1993and further renovated recently.

Several of these landmark buildings are illustrious examples of neo-Gothic architecture. Many years later when I was accompanying Sir Robinson, the noted British economist, from the airport to Taj Mahal Hotel, where he would stay as a guest of Tata group, he was very happy to see the Flora Fountain/ Hutatma Chowk, saying that it looked exactly like London.

I walked across the High Court and the Central Telegraph Office (CTO) building, passed by the 'holy' well of sweet water named after Bhika Behram constructed as early as 1725, between the Cross and Azad Maidan, leading to the crowded Churchgate station – a box type new building next to the magnificent head office building of Western Railways.

I heard about the flowing stream of humanities rushing in unison to board their respective trains to reach home from Churchgate station. I witnessed this after several weeks by climbing to the terrace of the Churchgate building, where there was a wonderful restaurant run by Western Railways. Reaching there one evening little before 5 O'clock, I saw the most mind boggling sight of my life – literally a huge, endless stream of human beings, both males usually dressed in dull white and females in psychedelic colors, soundlessly walking fast towards Churchgate station. They disappeared into the two subways leading to the platforms of the station. Every three minutes a train either departed or arrived on an average. Reaching the control office of the upper floor, I also witnessed how people jumped into the speeding train even before it fully stopped!

I thought that when I would be going home in the evening I would also be just one, a new one added today, to the millions of people rushing to go home. Every day quite some new persons were added to the existing about 5-million local commuters of both Western (from Churchgate station) and Central (CSMT) Railways in Mumbai. Some people would also disappear from the stream though not every day.

In the morning the stream would be in the opposite direction, the commuters, literally in millions, come out from the station and walk sprightly to reach their respective offices. It goes on every working day in the morning and evening. On Sundays and holidays the entire area will be empty; there will be a few persons leisurely walking by.

I took my train, reached Bandra in about 20 minutes, walked across Hill Road, thinking all the time about Tapati. She must also be trying to get into an overcrowded bus from Gariahat to Jadavpur. Two soulmates are in two distant metropolis of the country, over 2,000 kms away. I was thinking how I should manage to get out of this mess.

My mind was moving deeply into all this and I realized that I overshot my right-turn on the Water Field Road for going to my PG accommodation. Since I had nothing to do going 'home', I walked ahead towards Band Stand. It is a beautiful, rocky beach, with waves hitting the rocks. On the left side of the road opposite the beach are rows of beautiful buildings where some film stars of Bollywood reside. There is also the historic Basilica of our Lady of the Mount, popularly called Mount Mary, where every year on the first Sunday after September 8, the birthday of the Virgin Mary, the feast is celebrated followed by a weeklong Bandra fair. Literally, thousands of people visit the Basilica during this time.

I stood there on the rocky beach for quite some time, looked at the evening sky, which was gradually taking a haunted shape with the twilight glow. Stars are slowly coming up one by one, then suddenly many of them. Darkness enveloped the sky and the sea. Mild waves are breaking on the rocky beach. One face is coming up in my mind. Tears, tears started flowing out. I got up after half an hour and walked up to Alameda Park. After having a bath, I realized that I would have to eat. I was hungry. I went to the nearest second grade Udipi restaurant on Pali Hill Road. Udipi is a town in Karnataka; people from Udipi run the popular eateries, serving South Indian dishes all over Mumbai.

My room was comfortable, well furnished. From the seventh floor window, I could see the Alameda Park. Looking at the soft lights of the park, my mind travelled to Pushpa Kuthi. The yellowish dimly lit view of Alameda Park of Bandra moved my mind to the surroundings of Pushpa Kuthi at Garia. From the large window in the south of our fourth floor flat, the vast empty space looked pitch dark at night. I imagined that I was standing on the narrow balcony of Pushpa Kuthi. Tapati was on the side holding my shoulder. I could inhale a light fragrance from her hair. The night was very breezy. One of two tiny dots of lights was seen at the distant horizon. At night, there was a dimly lit bulb in the courtyard that created a hole in the darkness. Beyond the wall, there was a row of coconut trees. In the breeze, they were moving their leafy head from one side to the other. Their shiny leaves were slightly visible in the soft moon light. The sky was bluish dark and clear with floating whitish clouds sometimes passing over the three quarter full moon. The soft moon light created a romantic set up.

Suddenly, a soft and melodious tune started coming from below. I came back to my reality – I was not in Pushpa Kuthi, I was in Honeycomb building at Bandra West looking at Alameda Park from my large glass window. Holding back tears, I decided to fight my destiny, our destiny. I wrote a long letter to Tapati. Our struggle in life had just begun.

I switched off the light. Rays of light from outside entered my room through the Venetian blinds and with the soft melodious tune from Anand Bakshi's flat down stairs, it created a beautiful paranormal environment.

Shaping Up of a Corporate Economist

Many passengers are asleep. Some are half-heartedly watching movies. The majority are Indians. Elderly and middle aged people outnumber the young. I wonder why so many people go to America and what they do there! Everyone must have a story to tell.

The next day I entered the office wearing a full-sleeved shirt, discarding my suit, amidst some laughter and clapping. Some of my colleagues had a bet on whether I would go to work on my second day wearing a formal dress or not. The winners were clapping.

Pendse welcomed me in the DES in a formal way. He told me that the practice there was that a young economist would be attached to a senior economist who would play the role of a mentor. He told me that I would have to be involved in doing the work for J.R.D. Tata, the Group Chairman, whose interests were wide, including national and international issues. J.R.D. Tata (1904–1993), the doyen of Indian industries expanded Tata Group's business in a big way. He is a well-known personality because of his wide variety of activities and interests. Pendse explained to me about the meticulousness of J.R.D. Tata and his wide areas of interest. He also assured me that an intelligent person like me would soon learn the required details.

Leafing through JRD's (as he was called in Bombay House) file, I was flabbergasted. The file was about two inches thick, packed with notes and papers. The very first 'Note' from the DES in the file was a cyclostyled note on Energy Crisis. The 10-page note had numbers of handwritten correction almost on every page. The title, 'Energy Crisis' was corrected by adding a large font 'The'. I thought of using the phrase 'star studded' for those corrections. At the end, JRD wrote, and I remember almost word by word, "an otherwise excellent note has been thoroughly spoiled by…"

I read the note twice and carefully noted the corrections. I took a pledge that my note must not be returned with such 'star-studdings'. I saw a number of letters from very top-notch people who wrote to JRD Tata and his replies. I went on pondering over it to organize my mind to do a neat job.

At lunch, I tested my first Parsi preparation of *Patra ni Machhi* (half of a large pomfret with soft spices (wrapped in banana leaf and baked), rice and thick *dal*. That was my first full meal in last five days. It tested heavenly! I paid just Rs 3.50 at the subsidized rate. Later, I became a great connoisseur of Parsi cuisine like *chicken farcha, dhansak, sali mutton and sali boti*.

On Friday morning, I received two copies of '*The Economist*' Newspaper about which I have already mentioned. I was told that I would have to mark the copies every Friday before five p.m., one for J.R.D. Tata, and the other for N.A. Soonawala, Director, Tata Sons Ltd, for their weekend readings. Soonawala was the financial expert in the group. I came to know later that many senior directors and executives do serious readings of topical books, journals and business magazines. I was happy because I would be able to read '*The Economist*' newspaper regularly.

Gradually, I got accustomed to the working of the DES. An assignment arrived from Jamshed J. Bhabha, Chairman of our company, TSL and a director of Tata Sons Ltd, the holding company of the Tata Group companies. He was the brother of Dr. Homi J. Bhabha, the 'father of India's nuclear program'. J.J. Bhabha, I heard later, was in-charge of art, culture and publication related activities of the Tata Group.

My first assignment was to write a quick note on Walter Lippmann (1889–1974), the noted American writer, journalist, commentator, twice winner of the famous Pulitzer Prize. His syndicated column, '*Today and Tomorrow,*' was published in many newspapers. He interviewed Nikita Khrushchev in 1962. He also got the highest American civilian award, 'Presidential Medal of Freedom' in 1964. He was the 'Father of Modern Journalism' as well as 'the most influential journalist' of the 20th century.

It just happened that I had read about Lippmann before and had some understanding about the man and his works. Vinu Bhai was my senior economist to provide guidance on this assignment. We had a discussion and I told him about my understanding about the man and his works. I re-read some of his books and some articles on his works, and prepared my note. It went to J.J. Bhabha and after about a week, I heard that he liked it.

I realized that my wide range of reading was becoming useful. I heard later that because of the exposure to various areas they decided to recruit me in the Tata's Think Tank. I thought, however, that I would have to concentrate to do a more systematic, organized and careful reading and contemplation as well as develop specialization in certain fields.

My next important assignment was for JRD. Three books were written by Ferdinand E Marcos (1917–1989), President of the Philippines for a quarter century from 1965 to 1986 of which 10 years were under martial rule (1972–81). The books were: '*National Discipline: The Key to Our Future, 1970*', '*Today's Revolution: Democracy, 1971*', and '*Notes on the New Society of the Philippines, 1973*'. These three books, autographed by President Marcos himself, were presented to JRD, with a letter forwarding the books, and requesting for his comments.

Marcos was a brilliant student and excelled in sports like boxing, wrestling and swimming. He ruled the Philippines as a dictator, was allegedly involved in embezzlement and other corrupt practices. He wrote 12 books. My assignment was to draft a brief review of those three books for facilitating an appropriate reply, acknowledging the receipt of the books as well as making some comments.

It was quite a challenging task for me, who had just joined the DES. The note had to go to J.R.D. Tata, who became a legend in his lifetime. However, I was quietly happy.

Those were not the days of PCs, laptops, smart phone, internet, Google search and all that. We had to find printed reading materials. It was not easy to get the latest ones. After doing some reading and research, I prepared a draft, and, read some more literature on Marcos, and I left it for a day. I improved it the next morning and sat down quietly to re-write the piece by my hand carefully.

I titled the note, 'The Tall Shadow of a Short Man'. I submitted the piece to Pendse a few days before the deadline. The next day Borwankar told me that my note had gone to the Chairman's office. I was happy because I did not have to go through further hassles.

I prepared the text remembering the purpose that it would facilitate writing a reply, with some relevant highlights and brief comments. I mentioned the highlights of the key points made by Marcos in his three books in brief and added my observations. I indicated that the basic issue arising out from the books under review was a concept of 'Dictatorial Democracy' (my words).

Even after four days, I heard nothing. On the fifth day, Pendse called me. He gave me back my Note, which had come back from Chairman's office. There was no 'star studding' on the note. No comments either. Finally, he smiled and told me that I would have to prepare a single page draft reply from J.R.D. Tata to President Marcos. He told me that there had to be some polite appreciation of the President's views, yet not agreeing to his thesis. I was relieved.

I made a couple of drafts and thought through how it could be more pertinent. Eventually, I finished the draft on my second day before lunch, got it typed and sent it to Pendse. After a few days of suspense, a copy of Chairman's reply to President Marcos came to me. I was happy to see that except some small editing, my draft was largely accepted.

The following week, at 5 O'clock in the evening I had to go to Dr. Freddie A. Mehta's office on the right corner next to our office. He was a brilliant student. He did his PhD from London School Economics in International Economics. He was the first Tata Administrative Service (TAS) officer. JRD thought that a talented cadre of service like the Indian Administrative Service should manage the Tata Group companies. Thus, TAS was created and TAS presently is a much sought after placement option for bright MBAs.

Dr. Mehta was the second EA of the DES, created at the instance of JRD as early as in mid 1940s. JRD thought that India would be Independent, businesses would grow and it was imperative that the corporate executives would need to get a clear idea about economic and business environment. Hence, there was need for corporate economists.

They would grow from the DES. It was really a great perception and initiative. He was a visionary in the true sense.

While on this, I must say that even today majority of Indian corporate sectors do not have economists in their team. They do not even know how to engage economists. It is true that engaging corporate economists was not required during the control raj when a clever chartered accountant and lawyer could have managed the show. Yet the perceptive JRD established the DES as early as the mid 1940s.

Y.S. Pandit was the first head of DES. Dr. Mehta succeeded Pandit. When Dr. Mehta moved up in the organization, Pendse joined as EA. I was recruited a couple of years after Pendse's taking over. However, I realized that on economic issues, the last word on critical economic issues had to come from their *Apro* (their own) Freddie.

When I went to Dr. Mehta's office, Pendse, Vinu Bhai and Borwankar were already seated in his office. Pendse introduced me briefly and excused himself out. Dr. Mehta nodded and smiled at me and started a monologue on certain economic issues. The meeting for my 'introduction' to Dr. Mehta was over after half an hour of Dr. Mehta's monologue on certain economic issues! There were quite some sparks in what Dr. Mehta said. I decided to follow up those points. My learning of the practical aspects of economics began then.

Time moved on. Communication with Tapati was mainly through written letters. Sometimes I would call her at her National Atlas office from DES after taking permission for making a brief personal trunk call. Sometimes on Sundays, I would go to the Central Telegraph Office (CTO) across the fountain to book a trunk call (as long distance domestic telephone calls were called those days) to talk to her. Booking a call, waiting for the connection, and cancelling the booking if the connection could not be made used to take the larger part of Sunday. Today's instant and inexpensive communication was beyond our dream in those days.

My work moved on. The Jaisukhlal-Hathi Committee Report on Indian Drug and Pharmaceutical Industry was released in April 1975. It was landmark in the country's pharmaceutical industry. I had to draft a DES note on the recommendations of the report for circulation to directors. I decided to do it in the style of the DES notes, brief, focused, pragmatic and with appropriate critiques as well as comments. I spent the Saturday and the Sunday to read, think, write, re-write and finalize the draft. Pendse approved the draft and the note was circulated. I guess, I entered the DES core.

Almost every day Dr. Mehta used to walk in, making some comments aloud on certain issues. He addressed his comments usually to Vinu Bhai. That was his practice. The fact was that Vinu Bhai had a very wide reading habit; his understanding of certain areas of Economics was both wide and deep unlike others. While returning to his office next door one day, Dr. Mehta waved me to come with him.

Once inside, he asked me about my background, my reading habits and my views on a number of issues on Economics and politics, about capitalism and Communism and China.

I was sure that he had some idea about my background. I wondered whether I was attending yet another interview. While answering him, I mentioned about my participation in the Leslie Sawhney Program and all that. There was also a discussion about Lord Keynes' works, the Great Depression. Keynes' suggestion for increasing public expenditure to create net assets, leading to employment generation, growth and the New Deal that followed, the market-oriented approach with powerful intervention by the Government as and when necessary, the essence of the Bretton Woods architecture, etcetera, etcetera.

He listened, with frequent comments and questions. At the end, he smiled and said, "Good, thank you." I went out wondering what the purpose of the long meeting was. There must be some purpose.

After lunch, Dr. Mehta went to Pendse's cabin, called me and gave me an assignment, which was confidential. He explained the brief outline of the project, asked me to read all necessary materials, prepare a detailed work plan and points to be covered within a week. I would work under his direct supervision. He also told me that if I could come to office on some Saturdays, then he would sit with me to discuss the assignment. That was one polite way of ensuring that I would go to office on Saturdays. At the end, he cautioned me, "Nobody knows what you are doing."

The assignment came from the top level of the Government of India. Such projects used to come to DES from high levels of the Government when an independent or neutral view was required before taking some important decision on a particular issue. The present assignment was very sensitive in nature and hence the secrecy.

I worked for over a week on research and prepared a draft work plan. Dr. Mehta was there on some Saturdays. Borwankar and a couple of others used to work regularly on Saturdays. Dr. Mehta was fond of Bombay's well-known *Batata Vadas* (round – shaped and deep-fried potato chop, one of Mumbai's popular snacks). There was a good restaurant called Pyrkes in fountain in those days. He took us to Pyrkes for *Batata Vada* and coffee some Saturdays.

Within three weeks, I completed the draft, discussed with Dr. Mehta, and Borwankar on the side, revised and finalized it before typing. Dr. Mehta added a short covering note with his signature. For obvious reason the note was typed on plain paper, not on office letterhead. He smiled and nodded to me and left with the papers.

I had no idea where it was going and for what purpose. I got to know after about one month. He told me the full context one day that certain important decision was to be taken at the top level of our Government. The note that I prepared under his guidance was very useful to facilitate the decision, whatever that might be. Great! I was happy. I promised him that I would never reveal the details.

Thereafter, I worked for, and with him on two separate assignments, India's agriculture and technology transfer, prepared for two separate international seminars. The projects helped me to widen my horizon and add to my knowledge.

Working on Economics-related issues for JRD was a different experience altogether. For instance, J.R.D. Tata was a member of an advisory body to Chase Manhattan Bank. He was the only person from the Third World. Henry Kissinger was the head. Those days Chase organized two seminars in a year, one used to take place in the USA, and the other in Europe. The theme of the seminar used be futuristic, sometimes far-fetched and scenarios building types. JRD would speak on the theme immediately after Kissinger.

The process of the work started a couple of months before the event. I prepared the first draft carefully. Pendse and concerned senior members read and discussed the draft. Then the revised draft would go to JRD. He would also give his views in a meeting. Based on all that, I would prepare, in consultations with seniors, a revised draft. That would come back with many queries and comments from JRD. After several such rounds, JRD himself would give a dictation on the subject of his talk. Revising his draft was the most sensitive and therefore, the most difficult part of the job for obvious reasons. That would go for a couple of rounds before the contents of the speech were finalized. He would not read out the prepared text. He would speak. JRD was a very meticulous person. Working for him widened my knowledge base.

Apart from the speech, the other part was to prepare the possible or likely questions that could be asked and prepare answers to those questions. After the event, the printed copy of his speech would again be revised and improved, and then it would be published as a Tata booklet with a snow-white cover with titles printed in red. One had to be on one's toes until the whole process was over. It was difficult to run through such a long process. However, it helped me to learn a lot. It gave a polish to my career.

One interesting anecdote I must mention about JRD. Once some papers were sent from DES to him where the stapling was done in an inappropriate manner. JRD wrote back in a step by step way about how one must staple pages – stapling should be done on the left top of the sheets of paper at a 45 degree, keeping sufficient distance from the left and right sides, so that the paper can be turned easily. Besides, after stapling, check the reverse of the paper and blunt the sharp points of the pin – the reader's fingers must not get pricked by the pin ends.

I was also closely involved in working for Naval H. Tata (1904–1993), Deputy Chairman, Tata Sons Ltd, the holding company of the Group as well as responsible for the then three electricity companies and four textiles companies. He was a different personality compared with J.R.D. Tata. He contested the general election, but lost. He was a great lover of hockey, was the President of Indian Hockey Federation for 14 years, when the India team won Olympic gold medals in 1948, 1952 and 1956. He was the father of Ratan N. Tata, who succeeded JRD as Chairman of the group. What many people did not know was that he was a member of the governing council of International Labor Organization (ILO) for over three decades. Besides, he presided over the Employers' Federation of India from 1959 through 1984. He was a member of the labor panel of the Indian Planning Commission in 1966. He was a warm person, smart and an intelligent communicator.

He had to deliver talks in the meetings of the governing body of ILO, seminars as well as meetings at home and abroad. Working for him, of course, was challenging but it was very direct and ended in just about a couple of rounds. We had to prepare the initial draft on the given themes, often a set of six related topics. He would read the draft; suggest some changes and revisions. The revised draft would go to him. Usually that was the end from our side. The papers would come back from his office with many papers and documents after his return from the trip and generous thanks.

I had worked with several senior directors in the Group. Each one was different from the others. Their style of work and field of expertise were also obviously different. It was a great learning for me to be associated with those important corporate leaders. I shall write about some of them later in the book.

Talking about our internal works in DES, working for and with Pendse was a different experience compared with Dr. Mehta. Pendse would do a lot of hard work in organizing a paper, would get many of us involved and try to get the best out from everybody and he was extremely meticulous in finalizing the report. His eyes would not miss a comma.

Dr. Mehta's approach was different. His knowledge base was deep, horizon wide and his insight on economic issues was focused. He was a fast reader, once he organized his thought on the subject, he would give a long dictation to his secretary Nargis in the presence of those of us working on the job. We would run through the pages carefully, draw his attention in case of doubt. Then he would take a final look and suggest some changes. Then we took care of the final paper.

Working with different personalities helped a greenhorn like me in the field. Such exposures widened my horizon and helped me to organize my own method of delivering the job.

Grown up in West Bengal, the base of left-centric ideologies, I did not carry any baggage at all. While working for and with some of the top industry leaders, in the Tata Group I realized that the group's vision and philosophy was humane. They were different. The major stakeholder of the Group – presently, over 66% of the shares of major Tata group companies – are owned by Tata Trusts, which recycle the profit back to the society.

They run the business efficiently, but they are not profiteers. Besides, the Tata Group introduced many welfare measures like eight–hour work, equal pay for both men and women, leave with pay, provident fund scheme, medical aid, accident benefits and education of kids for industrial workers much before those were made mandatory by legislations of the country.

It is from the Group's Economic Think Tank that I got my grounding and was able to take off – if I may say so humbly.

CHAPTER 27

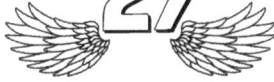

Living Together – At Last

Four days of Diwali holidays are welcome. It is an India wide festival of light, fireworks, purchases of dresses, jewelries, cars and flats. It is a celebration of life. It is worship of the goddess of wealth, Lakshmi in some parts of India. But in Bengal, this is the time for the worship the goddess of destruction of evil and darkness, Kali. It is a time when everybody wishes everybody a long and healthy life, happiness and prosperity. It is a great time for business. Sales graphs move up sky high before and during Diwali, and quickly plunge far below the base level immediately after Diwali.

Tapati came to visit me for about two weeks in June 1975 and we had a great time. After my office hours, we used to move about the great city of Mumbai. The experience of watching the sea – the vast sheet of Arabian Sea stretching up to the horizon – moving across the semi-circular and long Marine drive, viewing the beautiful Queen's Necklace in the evening, walking on the Hanging (Kamala Nehru) Garden and the Shoe House was a great experience. Riding a decorated Victoria was thrilling. We went to see the beaches of Mumbai – each one is different. The beach at Dadar looked longish but dirty. The Band Stand at Bandra is the only rocky beach. Juhu beach is long and semi-circular, sandy and full of activities. It was great fun watching kids riding horse and camel, riding the merry-go-round, playing games, people going almost knee-deep in the water, eating junk food and cold drinks like Mumbai's favorite *Kala Khatt*a from dozens of eateries. Watching the Sun setting by the horizon of Juhu beach was a serene experience.

Versova beach is sandy, longish and usually not crowded. It is beautiful. Aksa beach off Madh island is semi-circular but very treacherous because of the under current, every year some young men are drowned because they go swimming violating the 'danger' notice. For senior Tata executives there is an exclusive beach resort on the Aksa beach. We went there several times when I reached that level.

We went to Matheran, the Tableland, popularly called 'Hill Station', at an elevation of 800 meters above the sea level on the Western *Ghats*. Known as the 'forest on the forehead' of the hill, it gives a magnificent view down below as well as the surrounding circular peaks of the *Ghats*. We reached by a toy train, a distance of 90 kms from Mumbai and 20 kms by toy train from Neral station. The roads were made of red laterite soil and no automobiles were allowed as it was an 'eco-sensitive zone'. There were 38 'points' from where we could view the wonders of nature. We visited some points, not all. The Panorama point provided a 360-degree view of the *Ghats* and the ground below at 800 meters. It gave a wonderful feeling of happiness.

I had heard people in Mumbai did not usually invite new comers at home for lunch or dinner, they entertained guests in restaurants. However, our experience was pleasantly different. Vinu Bhai invited us for a sumptuous Gujarati lunch. Sunil Bhandare, several years senior to me in DES, and Lata Rele, both Maharashtrians, invited us for hearty dinners. We greatly enjoyed the treat given by friends from DES.

We also visited Tapati's elder cousin Capt. D.M. Chakraborty, Doli da as he was addressed by his pet name, and his family – his wife Rani and kids Joya and Samu. Doli da, former Wing Commander of the Indian Air Force, opted to become an Air India pilot. They were very hospitable.

The time of Tapati's first visit was mid – June when Mumbai's famous monsoon had already hit. It was raining continuously for a few days. We enjoyed the rains, walking out in the rain with knee-deep water on the roads. It was a new experience. Then she had to go and we separated again with tears in our eyes.

I visited Calcutta during Durga Puja time and had a joyous reunion with the family and relatives. My in-laws took affectionate care of me. It was a food festival every day. My father-in-law went to the market for different types of fishes or meat. My mother-in – law was a great cook. After four or five days of great time, I had to leave.

We managed with such occasional visits for quite some time. On one visit to Calcutta, my father-in-law fell ill. After his initial treatment, I had to return to work.

In the morning of July 25, 1978, I received a phone from Tapati that he was no more. She was profusely crying. I went to Calcutta to attend the rituals. While travelling in the train in an unreserved and crammed compartment, I remembered my first meeting with him in the Writers' Building. After our marriage whatever little opportunity we had to interact, we did converse about politics, literature and many personal things. I gave him the book by Aleksandr Solzhenitsyn, who got the Nobel in literature in 1970, 'One Day in the Life of Ivan Denisovich'. The book created quite some disturbing ripples in his Leftist mind. In the post – partition India, he was a sad man internally, but he maintained his pride and dignity. I respected him.

Several Left leaders and former freedom fighters maintained contact with him. Often they used to visit him for discussions, seeking his views and advice. The Jyoti Bose Government of West Bengal posthumously honored him as a mark of respect. The good gesture of the Government, however, caused considerable delay in settling his family pension. Tapati had to stay on to support the family. Her younger brother Shakti Prosad, a bright student, was studying engineering in the third year in the reputed Jadavpur University. Her immediate younger sister, Bratati had just completed her graduation. My mother-in-law, a very astute and practical person, took up the responsibility of the family.

I visited Calcutta many times for expediting the complex and time taking process of his pension. In those days, it used to take five to seven years to get the pension. Many retired school teachers and government employees died awaiting their small amount of pension. Eventually, with the help of Amal Roy, a member of the coordination committee of the State Government employees, the pension issue was settled. Amal was very respectful to my father-in-law.

During that time, I brought my Suniti aunt to Mumbai as a beginning for moving my family to Mumbai. She stayed with me for about a year. Tapati could not join me then. Being alone throughout the day, she was upset. An attendant we brought from Calcutta for my aunt was not of much help. My aunt was happy during weekends when some friends dropped in. As time progressed, she became adamant and wanted to go back to Calcutta. One particular theme she used to repeat was that she would like to be cremated after her death in the same crematorium in Kalighat where my grandmother was also cremated. She supported us with great care and at the same time, she was a stubborn person.

I had to take her back to Calcutta. Then my sister and her husband took her to their place in Siliguri. She stayed there for about two years. I had to again take her back to Calcutta. Where should I accommodate her? I did not have a place of my own in Calcutta. My mother-in-law graciously accepted her to stay with her. My sister-in-law Bratati and brother-in-law Shakti were also supportive and helpful. She happily stayed with them for two years.

Bratati arranged for my aunt's admission to Naba Nir, an old age home run by a reputed NGO. It is one of the best homes for the aged even today. Naturally, I paid the monthly fee, medical and other expenses. The home was close to my in-law's place. My mother-in-law also visited her frequently. My aunt was also very affectionate to Bratati and Shakti. She lived there comfortably until her death in 1993, at the age of 91. In my absence, Shakti lit the pyre as per our Hindu ritual at the time of her cremation. She had suffered a lot in life, so we never ignored her. Tapati, her mother, brother and sister treated her as one of their own family member. She died as a well loved person.

Life was difficult for the partitioned-affected elderly persons like my aunt. Their memory of life in East Bengal was more vivid; thus, their sorrow and misery were also very pronounced. Of course, she was very affectionate to Tapati, who was her family's *Bahu, and* always addressed her 'Ma'. She was also very affectionate to our son Sunny – the family's next generation.

Eventually, things settled in my in-laws' family. Bratati got a job in the same ministry where her father worked, a good gesture by the Government. Shakti was about to complete his engineering education. Eventually, Tapati resigned from her job and came to Mumbai by the mid 1979. She had to change her profession of a cartographer. She got a job as a Lecturer in a reputed college, established by Dr. Baba Saheb Ambedkar, in Mumbai and soon adjusted to the new lifestyle.

Tapati completed her PhD degree from Mumbai University in 'Retail Establishments', the only empirical study under Prof. Arunachalam, Head, Department of Geography, University of Mumbai in 1989. She pain-stakingly surveyed roads of Mumbai for her thesis work. Her thesis was published later as a book, the only technical book on the subject. She did several research projects under ICSSR, visited China thrice under the international exchange program for scholars under the partnership of ICSSR and Chinese Academy of Social Sciences (CASS) of China, published two more books, and prepared a number of technical papers. She actively participated in national and international seminars. Under her guidance, five students completed their PhD program; there are a couple of more in the pipeline. Apart from obtaining SAARC Fellowship in 2009, she also became Emeritus Fellow in Geography in 2013–15, and completed a research project on land administration and land use planning in Sindhudurg district, Maharashtra.

Her story of struggle for moving up in life and career is also the story of my generation. Tapati is also an example, born after a few years of the partition; her parents' family also suffered the pangs of post-partition life in Calcutta. Both of us are just two individual examples. There are many in my generation who had to struggle to move up in life and career. Each one has his or her story to tell. Our – the partition's children's – next generation started moving up further, attaining greater heights.

The company I worked for was Tata Services Ltd (TSL), which was a cost center. TSL was set up after the abolition of the Managing Agency System (MAS) around 1969. MAS was in vogue since the British days. Under MAS, Tata Industries Ltd (TIL) was a very powerful company as it was the managing agent for all companies promoted by the Tata Group.

The concept of 'Group' was there under MAS. However, when MAS was abolished, the Group concept was also gone. Thus, every company became an independent legal entity. That was done because of the high dose socialistic approach of the then Indira Gandhi government. The concentration of income and wealth in fewer hands was to be avoided for establishing equality!

The concern was that when a company was an independent legal entity, it might decide to operate independently. Thus, to sustain the Tata culture and ethos, TIL was converted into a kind of forum for the Chairmen/ MDs of the companies, erstwhile under the Group, where they could exchange thoughts and ideas. Besides, TSL was set up to provide common services to the erstwhile group companies. The services included our DES, PRD, legal services, Delhi office, medical services, labor relations and Tata Management Training Center (TMTC).

Thus, the cost of rendering those common services were to be borne by the major companies based on a formula. Being a cost center, DES' pay and perquisites were lower. However, I got promotion couple of times but the financial benefits were not much. The non-monetary satisfaction was that I had moved a couple of levels up and the work was intellectually satisfying.

During the initial period of five years, I had to shift my residence a number of times. Moving house had become a part of my lifestyle! I shifted from my paying guest accommodation to Santacruz East to share a flat with my friend Surhid.

One evening at Doli da's place, I met his brother-in-law Wing Commander Shyam Java. Shyam told me that he had just taken possession of a small flat in a new high-rise building at Andheri West, opposite the then landmark Rajkumar Hotel; if I wished I could move in. I signed a Leave License Agreement for 11 months with him and moved in some time in 1977.

We stayed in that flat for over two years. Shyam decided to sell the flat for capital gains. He had two ancestral flats at Mahim. He offered the vacant one to us. Shyam was a good friend. It would have been difficult for us to find a place in Mumbai without his friendly gesture.

We moved to Mahim, close to St. Michael's Church, popularly named as Mahim Church. It is one of the oldest churches in Mumbai, constructed for the first time in 1534 by the Portuguese, rebuilt many times. There is a popular belief that if you visited the church nine consecutive Wednesdays (Novena), your wishes will be fulfilled.

Literally over 50,000 people belonging to different religions visit the church every Wednesday. I do not know how many people's wishes have really been fulfilled.

Our son, Sunny (Somshuvra) was born in 1980 in Nanavati Hospital, Vile Parle West, under the care of Dr. Shankari, a reputed gynecologist of the city. At that time, we were staying in Mahim. We felt ecstatic. My parents would have been happy, if they were alive. Tapati's father also would have been happy that his grandson had arrived. I was feeling elated being a father. Yes, I now have my next generation to move ahead in life.

During that time, Shakti also moved to Mumbai as an engineer in the Bhabha Atomic Research Center (BARC), a premier nuclear research organization of India. He stayed with us for about six years. He took good care of Sunny. That gave Sunny good company.

In the weekends, Shakti's friends used to drop in to have the 'feel' of home – away from home. They were bright engineers just appointed at BARC and its outflows. Sunny also had a great time with them. He immensely enjoyed their smart company. Playing and mixing with mature boys helped him to grow.

Almost every evening at around 6 p.m., he had to be escorted by Tapati to Mahim station to receive me. That was the happy union of the small family in the evening. He would jump on my arms seeing me getting out of the train. He would babble many sweet things as a kid would say. He always would have a small list of items to buy. He must have them all.

He was like a night watchman, in his early years. Sleeping largely in the day and waking up in the night. By 9 O'clock in the evening, his eyes would light up. Sometime in the midnight if he had heard the honking of the BEST bus, he had to take a ride. His favorite was the red colored double decker trailer buses. Because of our frequent visits and rides on those buses, conductors and drivers became very fond of him. Having a horse ride on Dadar sea beach on a rainy day, he would insist on bringing the horse home, because it would otherwise catch a cold.

During that time we realized that we needed a relatively stable residence to stay – more so because of his schooling. I took up the issue of my accommodation with my company. They considered my request and allocated a flat in Tata Housing Center (THC), Andheri West. In June 1984, we moved in to THC where we stayed for almost two decades.

The location was very convenient for all of us. There were two large playing grounds in the housing estate. It was great for the kids. In the housing facility, there were not too many hierarchies maintained among residents. A number of sports and cultural activities were organized. For growing up kids, the place was a paradise.

Som studied in St. Xavier's School, Vile Parle from Junior KG to 10th standard. He was a bright kid, interested in sports and games at the same time. He played football as a goalkeeper, representing his school in the junior division, taking part in Mumbai's well-known Bipeen Memorial Tournament as well as in the inter-school league. As a goalkeeper, he made his name in the school circuit. School principals used to approach me to transfer Som to their schools.

He played in the popular Giles Tournament of cricket of Mumbai where many legendary cricketers of Mumbai played when they were school kids. He enjoyed playing all those games. At the same time, he performed excellently in academics.

In the school campus, stands a catholic church established in 1868. There is an old banyan tree overlooking the church. Initially, the school started under this tree in the early 1880s. The tree still stands there. It reminded me of the other banyan tree of my life in Simlagarh.

I was closely involved with the activities of the school as vice chairperson of Parent Teachers Association. As PTA member, we took care of the school's large playground and built up the football team. We introduced a midday meal scheme for students from lesser well-off families. The principal selected names of such students quietly. We contributed money to the school canteen, also quietly, for supplying food and snacks to those boys. From the PTA, we stood by the school authorities for whatsoever support they needed from us.

Principal Father Peter Paul Fernandez was a wonderful person. He was a music lover and could make you absolutely relax or dose off by talking for 10 minutes! Teachers took great care of students. Vice

Principals Pinto Sir and Julie Madam (junior section), Maira Madam and Lolekar Madam played a significant role in helping students grow up. Even after long years, they fondly remembered their students. When Som reached his 10th standard, he became chief prefect of the school because of his leadership quality. As parents, we felt proud.

Som's school teachers including Father Peter Paul were very loving and affectionate not only to him, but also to all other students. They reminded me of my teachers. They were wonderful persons – our children were safe in their hands.

Moving from secondary school, he completed higher secondary with excellent results and took admission in Topiwala National Medical College & BYL Nair Charitable Hospital Mumbai, popularly known as Nair Medical College, for his MBBS course.

Nair Medical College is one of the four reputed medical colleges of Mumbai. They are all public funded. It is a dream come true for bright students to get admission in any of these four medical colleges. These great institutions have been producing talented doctors year after year for many decades. Such public-funded medical colleges are there in some other metropolitan cities of India. There are eminent doctors who teach there and students are respectful to them. Som also respectfully remembers many of them. The kind of wonderful services they render to students and patients are remarkable.

Besides, there are many such public-funded higher education institutions like the IITs, IIMs and a number of others educational institutions. They played a vital role in the growth and development of the country. They have been paying back to the country many times more that the amount spent on supporting their education. I intend to take up this point later in the book. Besides, students from the public-funded institutions like IITs and IIMs have been attaining great heights abroad. Such students have been contributing hugely in the fields of education, management, medicine, engineering, IT services and finance. They are all products from the public-funded institutions of India. Many of them come back home, either permanently or occasionally, and continue to contribute financially or otherwise, including helping their alma maters.

Such public-funded higher and technical education institutes are stars of our country, they should be allowed to not only continue, but also grow.

Getting admission to the chosen medical hospital and colleges like Nair was obviously not an easy task in our country. We have seen some of our friends' children fail by just one mark. They had to go to second grade colleges. Som worked intelligently and hard. He decided early that he would study medicine, and only medicine. We did our best to help him.

He completed his MBBS successfully. He did not want to be a practicing physician and wanted to do research. So he moved to the United States for further education and research.

During that time, many people used to visit us. Our house was the weekend home for Shakti's friends. Many relatives and friends from Calcutta came to visit Ajanta – Ellora and Goa. The used to stay with us in between those trips. Iain and family as well as some of their friends were occasional guests. My students from Narendrapur also visited us. I heard from my aunt that guests were always welcome in our house in Hasial. We happily continued with the tradition.

CHAPTER

28

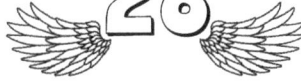

Moving Up the Ladder

I participated in the 12th International Business Forum, organized by the World Bank Institute and InWEnt, a German NGO, in October 2007 in Washington D.C. Som came to Washington and we had a wonderful sightseeing tour of the city. He drove me to New York. We had a great time together for a couple of days. I was happy to find him confident, focused and independent-minded.

Apart from our usual corporate work, we were closely involved in many topical areas of research, which needed timely attention of a think tank. I was deeply involved in many of those studies.

During the first half of 1980s, energy related issues; particularly renewable or non-conventional sources of energy became important. In DES, some of us developed certain degree of expertise in the field of energy studies, both conventional and non-conventional. I did a detailed study on the prospect of nuclear energy in India.

Pendse took part in several energy conferences abroad. I had to handle certain specific portions of the job. Over a period, I became interested to work in the field of energy economics. I did quite some coordinating job for Pendse's papers like getting them edited and printed in the new IBM typewriters, then very latest at the Tata Consultancy Services (TCS) office. Those were the days of doing 'cut' and 'paste' job literally by hand, slicing of the corrected typed words and sticking them on the manuscript pages. Then, we took photocopies in a very smart copier. Today, even the IBM typewriter, not to speak of Remigntons, cyclostyling machines and hand operated Facit 'calculators' must be huddling together for space in the museum.

Darbari Seth, a bright chemical engineer, educated in the USA played a significant role in establishing and developing Tata Chemicals at Mithapur. J.R.D. Tata selected Seth against the opinion of all other board members.[1] In fact, JRD had an insight in selecting young talents, having high potential to become business leaders in the future. Not only Seth, he selected several others of similar caliber.

Seth took the pioneering initiative for implementing the concept of 'energy conservation' immediately after the oil crisis of October 1973. In fact, under his guidance, Mithapur plant achieved more than 25% reduction of energy consumption. Eventually, other energy intensive Tata and non-Tata companies took up such projects. Today energy conservation is an essential component of sustainability initiative.

That apart, he inserted full-page advertisements several times in national newspapers pleading that India should manage with her own indigenous energy sources. I heard that he bicycled within the Mithapur plant campus to set an example.

I was involved in doing the groundwork, helping him with readings, data and preparing notes. I took part in discussions with him. Once I mentioned about the content of the advertisement whether it would be realistic to say that India should manage with her energy resources alone when the country depended heavily on imports. He told me with a smile, "Give me what I want, the way I want, I know what I'm doing."

Such exposures helped me develop some understanding about the applied aspects of energy issues. I started writing papers and articles on energy related issue, made presentations in seminars and published them also. Those were alongside my corporate work. During that period, I published a number of papers and articles on important economic issues in various magazines and economic newspapers.

Pendse and I jointly published a long article on the private sector in power in '*Commerce*' weekly in September 1983. Later, I wrote a paper on the need for a comprehensive power policy in later years. Forum of Free Enterprise (FFE) published and circulated it as a pamphlet it in October 1995. Incidentally, FFE is a non-political and non-partisan organization, established in 1956 to educate the public of India on free enterprise and democratic way of life.

Apart from the ongoing corporate work relating to various fields, the focus of DES research moved to 'privatization' related research and publications under the guidance of Pendse. There was not much understanding about the concept of privatization during the initial period in India. FFE organized talks on privatization for its members with a small entry fee. FFE invited me to deliver those talks and I conducted a number of sessions.

Moving the focus away from energy related research, Pendse took the initiative to work and explore the area of privatization; a concept implemented by Margaret Thatcher, Prime Minister of Great Britain during late 1980s. The work of researching and writing involved not only the need for privatization, but also how to go about it. I helped Pendse with the work and jointly published with him. I also worked with him on assignments for international organizations. In fact, DES became a hub of privatization studies in the country. It needs to be mentioned that we did these specialized projects along with all our regular corporate assignments.

I published a number of articles on privatization in newspapers and magazines. A lengthy cover story, '*Roaring Wave of Privatization in Developing Countries*' was published in the weekly magazine '*Commerce*', October 26, 1986. The Economic Development Institute, World Bank, reprinted and used that paper as a course material for the programs organized for senior government officials.

We moved from 'why' privatization to 'how to do' privatization. I was closely involved in working with Pendse on a project sponsored by an international organization to study how to go about privatization in a company-specific way.

While doing those studies, we also realized that the process of privatization should not be applied in certain key areas where vital interests of the large number of people were involved. Depending on circumstances, those areas of public interest, in my opinion, include public utilities like local transport, electricity, cooking gas, water supply, and certain services of education and health care measures. The list is illustrative.

There have been academic discussions on the so-called 'merit' and 'non-merit' goods. However, we must not lose our common sense in deciding what goods or services should attract subsidies and what should not.

In India, subsidies of various categories are paid from the Union Budget, about 14% of our GDP in 2014–15. There, of course, is a need for targeting subsidies so that poor are the beneficiaries, not the rich. Many countries in the world, even the USA, not to speak of the EU nations, do give subsidies to the deserving. Scandinavian countries in general and a number of West European countries have been providing generous subsidies to deserving cases. Some of these countries were known to be the paradise of welfare economics. Due to certain economic compulsions like the reversal of demographic pyramid and structural problems, there has been some reduction, but the flow of subsidy continues. In China, obviously the flow goes on in a big way even after the adoption of the 'socialist market economy'.

Certain key services like education and health should not be removed from the deliverance of subsidies, despite certain recommendations for privatizing them. Privatization of these two sectors would lead to huge increase in prices, which could not be affordable even by the middle class people. This will go against growth and development of the people of the country. For example, education and health are the vital services sectors that should regularly receive public funding. In fact, the required amount of spending repeatedly announced by the Government is that the desirable amount of subsidies should be 6% of GDP in real term for education and 3% for health care measures. The actual spending is meager.

While doing studies on privatization, we never thought privatization was a panacea to all ills. We took it up as a pragmatic approach to ensure that the public sector 'commanding heights', could perform better and earn a reasonable return on huge investments made from taxpayers' money. We desired that the public sector should not remain a milch cow for corrupt politicians, bureaucrats and power brokers. The management of the public sector must enjoy certain degree of autonomy, increase efficiency and productivity. Their balance sheets should be published annually. Privatization could certainly play a significant role in that regard.

M.R. Masani organized a seminar on privatization issues under the banner of 'Project for Education' at Agra in December 1988. On the second day of the seminar, I was seated next to Prakash Tandon (1911–2004), who was the first Indian Chairman of Unilever Hindustan Ltd, appointed in 1969. Later he became Chairman of Food Corporation of India. He was a formidable personality. He took me under his large and warm wings. While presentations were going on, he wrote brief and witty comments on slips of paper. He was not missing any point of the presentations. It was a fantastic capability, I thought. I read through the notes again and again later and understood what to say, what not to say, when one should stop talking, try to judge the mood of the audience and how to make brief as well as succinct comments. Despite difference of status and age, we became and remained friends for years.

He was fond of our Statistical Outline of India (SO), the popular pocket book of statistics, edited and published by DES. He also liked the popular small Tata diary in red color with a golden-capped pencil attached to it.

SO was a very handy source of data. It was very popular. I got to know that Indira Gandhi sent a note to Director General, Central Statistical Organization (CSO), the repository of India's macro-aggregates, enclosing a copy of SO, and asking how Tatas could publish such an up-to-date pocket book of processed data, largely using official data, and why the CSO could not publish such a useful book on time.

Many people did not know that SO was also a brainchild of J.R.D. Tata. He thought that people at the decision-making level would require processed data. He suggested to Y.S. Pandit, the first EA of DES, to do something about it. During the early years, the data sheets were cyclostyled and circulated. That was the origin of SO. Subsequently, the SO was printed as small pocket book annually and released on December 25. P.K. Sen handled the SO for a long time along with Mr. Kale and B.S. Gupta.

Later in my career, I took over the responsibility of editing and publishing the SO. We decided to make it a priced publication. At the same time, we continued to give complementary copies to people who mattered. Members of the Indian Economic Association might recall that we used to distribute complementary copies of SO to them. That raised interest in data use as well as the popularity of the S0.

Masani was invited to write a paper on Monopoly and Mixed Economy. I wrote the paper, '*Monopoly and Mixed Economy: What is Our Choice?*', which was published as a glossy booklet by Project for Economic Education. I presented the paper at a seminar on June 22, 1991 at The Taj Mahal Palace Hotel, Colaba, Mumbai organized by Masani. Pendse was on the chair. I was the only speaker and I was overwhelmed to receive such recognition from an astute person like Masani. I attempted to thank him, but he told me pointedly, "I knew you could do this. You will go a long way. Do not relax and be contented."

Sister Nivedita once wrote people should be driven by 'divine discontentment'. Humbly put, I have been following her advice. In my intellectual grooming, Masani played the role of a teacher and mentor. That did not mean that I had to agree with him on everything he would say. I did not agree with him on his strong rightist views. I told him that vast, diverse and poor country must follow the left of center approach in its economic management. He encouraged disagreement – as long as it was logical.

One important work DES used to do every year was the analysis of the Union Budget. Apart from the corporate work on the subject, we were deeply involved in helping Mr. N.A. Palkhivala for his famous budget speech organized by FFE. His famous annual budget speech had a humble beginning in a hall of small Green Hotel, Mumbai in 1958. Eventually, it moved over to the Brabourne Stadium, Churchgate. According to FFE, the number of audiences exceeded 100,000. It was a landmark event in the city. We had to do a lot of work for him.

My first introduction to budget analysis started in 1975 when I had just joined. I read a lot, listened carefully to discussions, saw with awe how under the guidance of Pendse and Vinu Bhai budget related assignments for Tata Sons directors and Group companies as well as Palkhivala were prepared. Sunil Bhandare, later my predecessor as Economic Adviser of DES, was an able deputy on those projects to Vinu Bhai.

Copies of the budget used to arrive by flight after mid night, distributed to senior directors and DES team immediately at their residences. Next morning by 9.30 a.m., the first meeting was held in EA's office, followed by a more detailed one later in the day.

For Palkhivala, a set of relevant notes on economy and business related issues were prepared well in advance. After the announcement of the budget, a number of discussions used to take place among DES team members and specific notes were prepared for him. On the third or fourth day after the budget, Palkhivala would address the audience on his interpretation of the budget.

I developed my understanding about the budget from internal discussions in DES, personal effort as well as guidance from Vinu Bhai and Bhandare. That the budget documents used to come in 12 volumes was not known to me; they are 14 in number today. I had a better hold of it the following year. Since then I was closely involved in the budget assignments of DES. Over a period, I started writing, publishing about it, gave interviews and participated in TV chats as already mentioned.

In the internet age, the DES budget work norm has obviously changed. After the announcement of the budget, the following morning every economic and financial newspaper would publish detailed company specific analysis on the impact of the budget. Individual companies also have their own team, their IT savvy experts to do the budget analysis job. The hassles of DES work of the old tech time does not exist now. Besides, on TV channels discussions go on before and after the budget. I also took part in daylong TV telecasts on the budget day for many years.

FFE was organizing budget talks in several places in Mumbai and its suburbs. The Reserve Bank of India (RBI) invited me for their seminar on budget analysis after a few days of the announcement of the budget during the late 1980s. Dr. Sandesara, a respected professor of Industrial Economics from the Department of Economics of the University of Mumbai was also present. He appreciated me in so many words, "Jiban, you have elevated yourself to such a height that I feel proud of you." This was the best recognition that I received. Humbly, I touched his feet.

When I moved up the organization, all activities of mine increased. One of the best complements that I received on giving talks on the budget came from our family friends, Mr. and Mrs. Aziz Jamadar. They were so appreciative of my budget talk that they used to travel to several venues in a day where I was giving those talks.

Nowhere else in the world, the budget discussion is such a lively festival. I was an active reveler of this festival.

As already mentioned, challenging assignments used to come from J.R.D. Tata. He had multiple interests and he pursued each one seriously. He regularly spoke in national and international forums on many subjects. He was a pro reformer in a pragmatic sense. He was very familiar with demographic issues. Reputed demographers used to visit and discuss with him. He was a keen advocate of family planning. His passion for flying was well known. He was fully conversant with aviation economics. He endorsed environmental causes. He was the doyen of India's industrialists, a legend in his lifetime.

I did a detailed background work for his paper on Tata Group companies' early implementation of the environmentally compatible initiatives. As usual, it went through the tumultuous route as already mentioned. The detailed paper, '*The Tata Approach to Ecology and Economic Growth*', was published under J.R.D. Tata's signature in the UNIDO journal, both in English and French in 1982.

Tata Group companies have been seriously engaged in taking care of the environment and the community right from beginning. The visionary founder of the group, Jamsetji N. Tata (1839–1904) wrote, "In a free enterprise, community is not just another stakeholder in business but it is in fact the very purpose of its existence."

Tata Trusts recycles profit gained from business to take care of the community and environment. Besides, individual companies have also taken up community development and environmental protection activities in their plant areas. The concepts of Sustainability and Triple Bottom Line (TBL) are of very recent origin. However, Tata Group companies have implemented both the content and spirit of the TBL concept since inception.

Dr. S.P. Gothoskar, an expert on funds flow analysis, Reserve Bank of India, came to DES to meet Pendse. On Pendse's suggestion, Dr. Gothoskar requested me to prepare an analytical paper on the estimate of poverty in India for the biannual conference of Indian Association for Research in National Income and Wealth (IARNIW) to be held in Chennai.

Incidentally, IARNIW was a forum of economists and statisticians employed in various government organizations like Central Statistical Organization (CSO) and National Sample Survey Organization (NSSO). The forum provided them the opportunity to critically interact on various academic and technical issues, take part in seminars as well as conferences and publish papers.

Alongside my regular corporate assignment, I prepared a detailed and critical paper on the estimates of poverty statistics in India. Dr. Gothoskar liked the paper and invited me to present the paper in the biannual conference of IARNIW at Chennai in 1988. I did the presentation in the presence of many stalwarts on India's national accounts and senior economists. They appreciated the paper from an economist from the corporate sector. I was made a member of IARNIW.

That gave me an opportunity to interact with a galaxy of the country's national income accounting experts and other establishments, academic statisticians and economists belonging to National Accounts Department (NAD) of CSO, RBI, several ministries and Planning Commission. I was surprised to know that many of those professionals with the government establishments were very competent experts in their respective fields. Many of them worked with international organizations. Our national account experts had been invited by smaller countries to build their national accounting system. I developed a lasting personal relationship with many of them.

A number of my papers on national accounts related issues were presented in seminars or conferences of IARNIW over the years and were published in the association's journal 'Income & Wealth'. Subsequently, I became a member of the Executive Committee of the IARNIW in 1992, the only one from the non-government sector. Reading my paper on poverty, George Rosen, a reputed American economist, wrote to me: "…probably this is the best piece I read on poverty estimates in India."

Chasing the 'Uncaged Tiger'

Two most important things that a pilot must learn are to skillfully handle take off and landing. However, landing is considered 'a bit more hazardous'. According to Beoing statistics, 18% fatal accidents occur during 'take off and initial climb', while 29% during 'approach and landing'. Our time is coming close for the second one. The mosaic of twinkling lights are visible below – the great city of Mumbai that does not go to bed at night.

The decade of the 1990s began with a number of radical changes in the Indian economy in general and Tata Group in particular. Our life and career also moved along with those unbelievably fast changes. Not that everybody was able to cope with those changes. I moved fast enough to understand and learn new dynamics and interpret complex analytics for presenting challenging deliverables of my job as a corporate economist.

J.R.D. Tata, who built the Tata Group companies with his visionary leadership, was Chairman of the group for over half a century from 1938, 'passed the baton' to a young Ratan Rata on March 25, 1991. A new era began in the Group.

The Indian economy moved over from the control regime to a relatively open and liberal economy to face challenges of globalization as well as the coming up of the overwhelming IT age. Those three new developments, along with the change of leadership in the Tata group, brought in considerable dynamics in our assignments in DES.

The Indian economy was in deep trouble, almost on the verge of collapse. The country was about to 'default' on its external payment. The deteriorating balance of payments (BOP) situation reached a critical stage by the late 1980s. The Gulf War of 1990 added to the BOP problem. Price of oil moved up further and availability was severely constrained. Overall imports declined by 27.5% in 1991–92 over the previous year. The oil import bill increased by 157% in the same year, while exports declined by 2%. The flow of NRI remittances reduced considerably. Being scared, NRIs, pigeons of happy times, withdrew $ 900 million from their external account deposit. The rupee was depreciating sharply. The foreign exchange reserves came down to a rock bottom level, $ 896 million on January 16, 1991, equivalent to less than two weeks of imports. The ideal situation for a developing country like India was about seven months of import cover. The credibility of the country suffered a great blow. The RBI could not get new credit lines from external agencies. All that was the recipe for a disaster; the country was about to default on its external payments.

The country had to transfer about 47 tons of gold from RBI vault in installments to the Bank of England and Bank of Japan to arrange bridge funding of $ 400 million. It was as humiliating as pawning your family jewelry to get some loan. Of course, India repurchased the gold when the economic situation improved.

Often many do not realize the seriousness of the problem of 'default'. The gravity of the problem would be clear to people if they apply their mind to the recent example of a 'defaulter' country, Greece. The Economic Survey, 1991–92 defined 'default' as: "A default in payments inevitably leads to a breakdown in credit availability and in normal payments arrangements. Suppliers become reluctant to sell goods and services and insist on advance payments through banks of their own country. Typically, this leads to severe trade disruption which in turn forces severe and prolonged import compression, and results in shortages, industrial dislocation, severe unemployment and inevitably, in very high inflation."[1]

The immediate need was to arrange for an emergency bridge fund of at least $ 2.2 billion from IMF. The economy suffered from low growth, high inflation and critical balance of payments situation as already mentioned. The abysmally low 'Hindu' rate of growth of GDP a little over 3% on an average per year continued for three decades up to the end of 1970s. During the 1980s, the rate of growth of the economy somewhat moved up to about 5% per year, the 'neo-Hindu' rate of growth. Prof. Raj Krishna coined the 'Hindu' rate of growth, a popular term. No wonder, there was acute poverty, poor infrastructure, both physical and social and robust regional imbalance – all symptoms of a dysfunctional economy.

The fiscal deficit of both the states and the union moved up to as high as 12.7% of GDP in 1990–91. That led to raising the internal debt of the government to a high 53% of GDP. The economy was about to collapse. Consumer Price Index moved to as high as 13.5%.

The political situation in the country was also unstable. There were two short-lived governments in India during 1990 and 1991. The V.P. Singh Government was in office only for 343 days from December 2, 1989 to November 10, 1990. The Chandra Shekhar Government, with even a shorter tenure – just 223 days from November 10, 1990 to March 6, 1991, followed. However, Chandra Shekhar had to resign because of the withdrawal of support by Rajiv Gandhi, leader of Congress Party, amidst the critical budget session. Support was withdrawn on a flimsy ground that two constables were seen to be near Rajiv's residence. They were suspected to be spying. President Venkataraman requested Chandra Shekhar to continue until the formation of the new Government after the general election.

Unfortunately, the Government could not announce the budget at such a critical time of the country's economy. That was a very politically unstable and economically critical time for the country. Indian democracy was in an ungovernable phase.

Madhu Dandavate, Finance Minister in V.P. Singh's short-lived government, had to negotiate with the IMF for arranging funding support to save the country from being a defaulter in external account, a precarious and humiliating situation for a country. India had to take recourse to the IMF and borrowed $ 666 million from the Reserve Tranche (RT) during July-September 1990.

Again, in January 1991, the country drew $ 789 million under the First Credit Tranche (FCT) and yet another $ 1,025 million under the Compensatory and Contingency Financing Facility (CCFF) of IMF. Thus, during the tenure of Chandra Shekhar Government, and negotiated by Finance Minister Yashwant Sinha, a sum of $ 1,814 million was drawn from the IMF. While negotiating the deal, the Government expressed its intention of applying for an upper credit tranche (UCT) later in the year.

The IMF sanctioned the first tranche of loan on condition that India would undertake economic reform in a step-by-step manner as per the standard norms of the fund.

To be precise, before the P.V. Narasimha Rao Government assumed office, $ 2,480 million worth of IMF credit had arrived in the country. Finance ministers, Madhu Dandavate and Yashwant Sinha, respectively, initiated the negotiation for the necessary IMF funding.

These two Finance Ministers, under the leadership of their respective Prime Ministers, took care of the critical economic problem by approaching the IMF for funding support, the only available option that any country would have under such a difficult situation. They saved the country from a humiliating situation of being a 'defaulter' on its external payments.

Such IMF funding for structural adjustment facility always comes with the 'conditionalities' of reform and restructuring of the economy. The 'conditionalities' have been derived from the principles of the market-oriented economic policy, with Government intervention as and when required, originating from the Bretton Woods Summit (about which more anon). These are applied to all countries that approach the IMF for funding support of this category to avoid being a 'defaulter'.

Most unfortunately, Rajiv Gandhi was assassinated on May 21, 1991. That was the third political assassination after Independence. Mahatma Gandhi, a frail person in physique, was assassinated on January 30, 1948. Prime Minister Indira Gandhi (married to Feroze Gandhi), yet another frail person in physique, was shot in close range by her own security guards on October 31, 1984. What an intolerant and cruel society we live in!

After the general election that followed, P.V. Narasimha Rao formed a minority government on June 21 1991, with Dr. Manmohan Singh as Finance Minister. In fact, Rao first sounded I.G. Patel for the position of Finance Minister but he declined. The name of Dr. Singh was the second choice. They had to do the follow up the process with the IMF initiated by the two previous governments.

The Rao Government, with Dr. Manmohan Singh as Finance Minister, after considerable negotiation with the IMF, received $2,546 million, of which $ 858 million was under CCFF and yet another $ 1,688 million under Upper Credit Tranche (UCT) worth of 'repurchase facility' from the IMF during the period July 22, 1991 through December 9, 1992 in several installments. Besides, it was also negotiated that $ 650 million might have to be taken under UCT in February and May 1993, in two equal installments.

Thus, before Rao Government came to office, the two previous Governments already obtained $ 2,480 million, or 49% of the total IMF funding. Over and above, the Rao Government arranged $ 2,546 million, in all a sum of $ 5,026 million. If the two UCTs were drawn as per the original understanding, the total amount would have been $ 5,676 million.[2]

The IMF apart, the Government had to approach the World Bank as well as Asian Development Bank for additional funding at different times during that difficult period

The predictable measures that Rao Government had to take as 'conditions' for availing the above mentioned loan from IMF for reforming and restructuring the economy followed soon. To begin with, the Rao Government had to devalue the Rupee in two installments in June last week and July first week, 1991, in all by about 20%.

There was an urgent need for macroeconomic stabilization, towards which a number of policy initiatives were taken on a moral equivalent of war. Dr. Manmohan Singh announced the budget on July 28 1991, followed by the release of the new and liberal industrial policy, 1991–92 in the evening.

I think it is appropriate to put certain historical details in their true perspective based on official record. These radical changes have taken place in our presence. As a corporate economist, I think it is important to give the readers a realistic perspective on the rapid transition of the Indian economy.

As usual, on the budget day we were in the office, listening to the budget, read out by PRD in Bombay House. Strips of teleprinter messages on the budget were also there. We could not believe what we had been hearing. The following morning we read both the budget documents and the new industrial policy, 1991–92. We pinched ourselves to feel that we were alive and not dreaming, whether we were reading the revolutionary announcement all right. It was extremely bold and revolutionary. '*The Economist*' cover-paged the India story, '*Uncaging the Tiger*', in later weeks.

The old and restrictive industrial policy based on Industrial Policy Resolution, 1956, as amended from time to time, was replaced at one stroke by a forward-looking straightforward industrial policy. The reservation of large number of major and core sector industries for the public sector 'commanding heights' was abandoned, with a few exceptions. At the same time, the 'license, permit and quota raj' was abandoned. The MRTP Act was amended, withdrawing the need for getting prior permission for capacity expansion and diversification. A policy of reform of the public sector units was announced.

An export-oriented policy was initiated providing certain stimulus to exports, considerably reducing stiff restrictions and regulations. A massive delicensing and simplification of imports procedure was introduced with import entitlement schemes such as 'Exim-scrips' and for export promotion, canalized items were reduced and streamlined. In fact, the highly restrictive export-import policy was simplified. The erstwhile 'red book' became the 'green book'.

Largely, the Industrial Policy was made simple and forward looking so that growth of industrial production could continue to increase, adding value to the economy such as employment and income. Foreign direct investment policy, financial sector and stock market were progressively introduced.

Rao, with Dr. Singh as his Finance Minister, took leaders of the industry into confidence and informed them about the need for implementing the economic reform in general and bringing competition as a large section of industrialists were not at all keen to compete at home or abroad.

Alongside, the PM himself managed the show from aside, sometimes pitting one political group against the other, navigating the path of the flight through several air pockets and conducting the show without being visible. He had to manage the given 'socialistic' mindset of politicians, Left-minded intellectuals, senior journalists, the protection loving Bombay Club industrialists – in fact, the entire system, which was habitually following the Nehruvian path.

Subsequently, Rao took the bold decision to select J.R.D. Tata and awarded him the highest civilian award Bharat Ratna, in 1992 in his lifetime. Perhaps, that was to send a signal to the country that industry did matter for the growth and development of the country.

While on this, I intend to mention that two recent books have separately brought to light that it was P.V. Narasimha Rao, who marshaled the process of reforms, and Dr. Manmohan Singh played his crucial role under the leadership of Rao.[3, 4] I am in full agreement with these two authors.

The reform produced encouraging results soon. The high peak rate of over 400% of import duty, with about 200% weighted average rate, was sharply reduced to around 15% in a step by step manner. Virtually, all items under 'quantitative restrictions' (QRs) on imports were gone. The economy started gradually opening up for foreign direct investment.

There was marked improvement in the external sector due to measures taken by the Government. For example, foreign exchange reserves moved up to almost $20 billion by January 1995, a huge gain from less than $1 billion in January 1991. The current account deficit came down from the unsustainable 3.3% of GDP to as low as 0.1% by 1993–94.

Because of the improvement of the economy, the Government decided not to approach IMF for a medium term extended fund facility. Instead, the government decided to make an advance repayment of $ 1.1 billion to IMF in April 1994.

Of course, the other reason for not withdrawing of the last tranche of loans and the decision for the pre-payment of the loan were for neutralizing the political heat generated by the opposition to the process of reform. Whatever was the reason, that was an appreciable and pragmatic decision. The overall rate of growth of GDP in real term moved up to the average of 7.5% during the post reform years.

Because of the achievement of that high rate of growth, India now has been growing at the highest rate of growth in the world. India is the fourth largest economy in the world; of course, a long distance away from China and the USA, with an estimated $ 9.4 trillion GDP on PPP basis in 2017. However, its per capita income on PPP basis is yet very small $ 7,200 as compared to China's $ 16,600.

China took a carefully considered conscious decision to introduce the market-friendly economic reform, maintaining the communist rule, under the visionary leadership of Comrade Deng Zio Ping in 1978. It experienced double-digit rate of growth for almost three decades. China, with an estimated $ 23.12 trillion GDP on PPP basis in 2017, has become the number one economy surpassing the USA's $ 19.38 trillion.

At the same time, it should not be forgotten that the USA remains the top country in terms of GDP on official exchange rate, with $ 19.38 trillion in 2017 (estimated), followed by China ($ 11.94 trillion) ranking second and India ($ 2.439 trillion) in seventh position.[5]

A large number of countries had to approach IMF for funding support at the time of their respective critical economic situation. For example, several leading Latin American countries, Russia and the UK and East Asian countries had to approach the IMF for help. In recent times, Greece and several PIIGS countries (Portugal, Ireland, Italy, Greece and Spain) had to approach the IMF for much higher amount of loans and tougher 'conditionalities'.

It is important here to point out that the process of reform in agriculture, the supporting leg of the economy, was not taken up for reform and restructuring in India. However, Comrade Deng Xiaoping introduced the liberal market reform deliberately, not under any IMF diktat, starting first with agriculture and then moving over to external and manufacturing sectors later. China's 'socialist market economy with Chinese characteristics' retained the communist party rule for the government. The role of the Red Army also remained dominant. He meticulously monitored the phase wise progress of the reform, which delivered high growth and development of the country and people. This is the unique Chinese model.

The most critical issue before our country today is, how and where these vast mass of growing poor people would be gainfully employed, and how they would progressively move on to the higher income trajectory in an ongoing way? The answer lies in finding an Indian solution, an Indian model of growth and development. It has to grow from our own soil – not to be copied from elsewhere – not from the former Soviet Union, not from China, certainly not from international institutions. Politicians, bureaucrats, technocrats and intellectual people of the country – all have to apply their minds in finding a viable Indian solution for the typical Indian problem. It is a tall order, easier said than done!

The second most important development happened via the global route. The multilateral trade organization, World Trade Organization (WTO), was officially born on January 1, 1995 after long and torturous deliberations of over eight years since the initiation the Uruguay Round of GATT in 1986 in Punta del Este, the last Round of the GATT.

The Bretton Woods summit of the nations was held in the USA in July 1944 attended by 46 representative countries, British India included. The summit concluded with the decision for creating three world organizations, International Monetary Fund (IMF), World Bank (WB) and International Trade Organization (ITO). Besides, the fixed exchange rate with $ 35 per ounce of gold was formalized.

The IMF and WB were set up by 1947. However, The USA did not approve the concept of ITO. The ITO was too liberal for the USA in those years. As a result, the treaty of General Agreement of Trade and Tariff (GATT) was signed in 1948 as an interim arrangement. To cut a long history short, WTO replaced the GATT with the consensus arising out of the Uruguay Round of GATT. The agreement was signed by 123 nations, India included, at Marrakesh, Morocco on April 15, 1994.

Thus, the WTO was born, with an agenda of liberal multilateral global trade in all products and services, providing rules of global business based on 60 Agreements relating to various items of trade. As on July end 2016, there are 164 member countries and 23 'Observer' countries – meaning that they are awaiting their entry.

Simply put, WTO is the only global organization dealing with the rules of trade in goods and services and trade related issues between nations based on the Agreements as have already been negotiated and signed by the member countries and ratified by parliaments, if necessary.

The introduction of the reforms process as well as the setting up of the WTO opened the horizon of Indian economy in a spectacularly large way. Major Indian industries as well as trade and commerce were progressively being reformed, restructured, re-engineered to face global competition both at home and abroad. Many large central public sector units were also getting modernized and restructured for the same purpose.

Yet another landmark development happened in the second half of the 1990s, i.e., the arrival of the information technology (IT) age! Gradually, we started getting computers in our office, replacing typewriters. All of us got training in handling computers. Each one of us got a desktop. Gradually, the circulation of DES notes was computerized, replacing the cyclostyling system. We got our handsets – the mobile phones – by 1997–98. India today uses more than billion handsets. Twenty years ago having a handset used to be a corporate privilege. The story of fast changing hi-tech gadgets from the Facit machines to desktop to laptop to smart phone, revolutionizing the social media is well-known. By the end of 1990s, we moved on a super fast track.

Life and work leaped sky high in the 'boundary less' world. Our assignments in DES also moved over to the new age with huge opportunities, convenience and high speed delivery mode. All this generated a huge opportunity for working in this process of reform and restructuring of the Indian economy in general and business in particular.

I became an active player in this grand orchestra.

Breaking the Frontiers

*I complete the immigration formalities and come out from the green channel.
Outside the arrival gate, hundreds of people – relatives and chauffeurs are
waiting for their friends, relatives and guests. I see Laxman, my loyal and
friendly help, waving. I wave back. It is time to go home.*

Three important developments made a sea change in the economy
and business in India: Reforming the Indian economy, challenges
and opportunities for taking active part in the 'adversarially' competitive
global trade and the coming of the frontier breaking information
technology age.

We in DES also wholeheartedly joined this spectacular endeavor.
These new opportunities changed our methods of working style. We
moved over to a high-speed style of communication, smart ways of
providing deliverables as well as reducing the time. These new activities
of our DES will also, inter alia, explain how the Indian industry in
general and Tata Group companies in particular moved ahead to face
global competition. It was like getting ready for the Olympic Games.

After immediate assignments in DES relating to the path-breaking
budget of Dr. Manmohan Singh and the new industrial policy, opening
a number of windows and doors of the economy was over, some of us
plunged into analyzing the deeper implication of the liberal economic
policy of India. I was particularly interested in taking this exercise forward.

Meanwhile, Sunil Bhandare was appointed EA of DES in 1993.
Bhandare was an old timer; he had an understanding about fiscal and
monetary theories and practices. He moved ahead with DES's regular
activities, with our support and involvement. We recruited some young
economists.

J.R.D. Tata, Chairman, Tata Sons from 1938 to 1991, for over half a century, expired on November 29, 1993 in Geneva. He became Chairman of the Group when he was a young man of 34 years of age. He inherited just 14 enterprises worth about $ 100 million. When he handed over the 'baton' in 1991 to Ratan N. Tata (RNT), the number of enterprises increased to 95 worth $ 5 billion. (Incidentally, the revenue of the Group increased to $ 100 billion in 2012 when RNT retired). All this expansion happened during the 'license, permit and quota raj'. JRD was an extraordinary leader.

With the arrival of the liberal economic policy, Ratan Tata had already plunged on reforming, restructuring and re-engineering the Group companies, focusing on core competences of the businesses within the group as well as bringing in massive organizational and leadership changes.

As result of both macroeconomic and enterprises level changes, our assignments in DES came into prominence. We prepared various types of notes on the impact of radical reforms and restructuring in the economy and business. New areas of study and interpretation of the emerging reality became the call of the day.

During that period, I single-handedly did an important assignment for Tata Exports, presently called Tata International. The assignment was on how to convert the company into a Japanese type of *Sogo Sosha*, unique trading companies of Japan like Mitsubishi and Mitsui Itochu, trading in large number of products all over the world. I visited many of their offices in Delhi. Those fiercely competitive companies created a scare among American companies during the 1980s. That assignment opened a new avenue of exposure and learning for me.

With the establishment of WTO in 1995, yet another gigantic dimension of assignments relating to impact analysis of global competition arrived. That became a new and fast growing area of specialization of DES as well as of mine.

The WTO provided rules of international business through its 60 Agreements. A company and its executives needed to have a clear-cut understanding about those rules of the game, if they desired to take part in the 'adversarially competitive' (Peter Drucker) global business. With my background of specialization in international economics, I devoted long hours in reading and understanding the complex WTO rules based on the Agreements. I also discussed, and networked with some experts from the Ministry of Commerce, apex chambers of commerce, some law firms and research organizations in Delhi, who started specializing on WTO related issues. I prepared a number of notes for our senior directors, Group companies as well as for publication.

That was an exciting period for the Indian economy. On March 19, 1998, Atal Bihari Vajpayee, a Bharatya Janata Party leader, formed a coalition Government National Democratic Alliance (NDA). The Vajpayee Government not only continued with the liberal economic process initiated by the Narasimha Rao Government, but also expanded it in many ways.

That was a period of events not only in the areas of the economy, but also in foreign policy, trying to improve Indo-Pakistan relations, combating terrorism and conducting the underground nuclear test – Pokhran II.

Prime Minister Vajpayee set up a number of committees with leading industrialists in various areas of the economy. Ratan Tata was heading two such committees with members from leading industry groups. The purpose for setting up those committees with leading industrialists was to suggest a pragmatic and implementable line of approach to that government.

All that gave us in DES a huge opportunity to work on critical issues of business and economics. I moved over to give my best by utilizing that opportunity.

Mr. R. Gopalakrishnan (RG as he was known in Bombay House), former Vice Chairman Hindustan Lever India (now Unilever Hindustan), joined Tata Sons as an Executive Director in September 1998. He took interest in DES's work.

With RG's close guidance, and the approval of Chairman, I took a lead role in organizing a full-day seminar on '*Making Tata Group Companies WTO Savvy – From Awareness to an Action Plan*' on November 18, 1999 in Mumbai. It was organized because of the imperatives of global competitiveness related issues arising not only out of the WTO, but also from the liberal economic reforms in general. The issue was how to make industry operations at company level compatible with WTO Agreements and the rules of the multilateral business.

I did a presentation on the draft action plan for the Tata Group companies. After my presentation, and interactions with the participating senior executives, it was decided to set up Tata WTO Cell in DES, headed by me as Chief WTO Officer. There would be WTO Cells at the major company level, headed by a WTO Officer, who would network with the group level cell. All that opened up a new and challenging area for DES and me to work on.

I took the initiative to prepare a blue print of the work to go ahead at the company level. There would be an Awareness Program on the complex WTO issues at the company level. I would have to prepare a customized presentation for about five hours, highlighting the issues involved for a particular company and its major products to company level executives focusing on their business. It was meant for 'manager to managing director' of the Tata Group companies.

After the WTO Awareness Program was completed, we would conduct a global competitiveness audit at the company and its major products level. We named the initiative as WTO Diagnostic Audit (WDA). RG was with us for organizing that work plan.

WDA was not at all an easy exercise. I and my small team of young economists worked on making the methodology perfect with a carefully constructed 'concept' paper and a detailed 'questionnaire' for organizing key operating data from strategic business unit (SBU) levels. We devised a rating mechanism, WTO Audit Rating Norms (WARN) – attempted to objectively assess the WTO compatibility, i.e., the degree and the level of global competitiveness of a company, based on a number of parameters. The emerging seamless market under WTO was akin to a 'curate's egg' – opportunities combined with threats. Therefore, companies needed to adopt an ambidextrous approach, capitalizing on opportunities and deftly tackling threats from WTO perspectives.

Finally, we prepared an Alpha Numeric Color Coded Matrix to score the company's preparedness for global competition at a particular point of time, and then provided a strategic path to move ahead. We closely discussed with RG in preparing all those intellectual properties.

Our WDA methodology received approval from competent organizations like Tata Business Excellence Measure (TBEM) and JRD Quality Values (JRDQV) as well as some other competent bodies.

For organizing the detailed process, my young and highly enthusiastic team members like Jahangir Engineer, Mongesh Suman, Raghabendra Katoti, Sarita Aiyer, Aruna Parimi, Tanvi Popat, Sudeepta Chaudhury and Dipankar Dey were closely involved with me. The young economists got a lifetime's opportunity to work and excel in challenging assignments and evolving to be competent corporate economists. Besides, there were Sobha, an enterprising librarian and Nalini, a research assistant. My secretary Rukhshana provided lifeline support. Humbly put, I got a lifetime's opportunity to conduct a challenging orchestra.

For doing the WTO related assignments for companies within the Group, it was decided at the top level that the DES would be paid from the Brand Equity and Business Promotion (BEBP) fund of Tata Sons Ltd, created from the royalty paid at varying rates by Group companies depending on their size. That helped DES, a cost center, to be financially independent.

We did a pilot WDA for five subsidiary companies of a major Tata company. That was appreciated by RG, the MDs of these companies and some other senior directors. On the advice of y RG, I made a presentation on the pilot WDA at a high-level seminar, participated by directors and top executives of major Group companies and the Chairman. Therefore, doing a successful presentation was of great importance for DES and me. By then I had been elevated to the position of economic adviser.

I was awaiting my turn. My heart was pounding so much that I could hear the sound of my heart beat. I started as a man possessed. Eventually, I spoke for about an hour, with frequent questions and interventions. When I was revealing the global competitiveness scores on the alpha – numeric color-coded matrix, there was a silence. I gave the numbers for all five companies, drawing inferences on each one of them and giving the strategic path and concluded my presentation.

Directors asked me a number of penetrating questions. There was a substantive discussion among directors. At the end, it was decided in the seminar that the WDA exercise would be done for all major companies, following the WTO awareness program. They congratulated me for the presentation. Subsequently, in the next Annual General Management Meet (AGMM), an important event of the group, the Chairman and RG made a mention that the WDA program would have to be done for major Group companies. A great opportunity – and a massive task – for us.

Incidentally, in the AGMM Chairman Ratan Tata's hour-long speech was the most important event. A small group of five of us was privileged to be in his small team to organize that job. The theme used to move from meeting to meeting before settling down to the crux of the presentation – seen from several dimensions like economics, finance and management for the diverse businesses of the Tata Group companies amidst the domestic as well as global perspectives. Permit me to say that Chairman did have a carefully articulated mind of a professionally trained architect – the traits of a hard taskmaster.

The work started in DES in full swing. Both customized company specific awareness program on global competitiveness via WTO route, to name one, followed by the comprehensive audit exercise. The WTO related assignments kept us absolutely worked up during the next three years. Of course, there were a host of other corporate assignments to be taken care of.

I personally did over 70 such company and product specific WTO awareness presentations from managers to managing directors of Tata Group companies. The duration of the presentation for one company was for about four to five hours. In all, a total number of 3,500 Tata executives participated in the workshops and became 'WTO Evangelists', to use RG's words. It was really a stupendous exercise. Because of those presentations across Group companies, I got to know a huge number of executives – a great reward for me.

The WDA exercise followed the company level presentation. A WDA team used to be composed of two to three economists of DES under my close guidance, along with two or three senior executives of the company. All of us in the DES put our heart and soul into those exercises. We did about 25 WDAs for over 15 different Tata Group companies for their major product lines.

For example, we did the WTO audit for Tata Tea. The DES team stayed in Calcutta for about a week, closely interacted with the designated senior executives of the company, collected data and information for the audit work and eventually completed the report after several rounds of revision under my close guidance and monitoring.

When the report was submitted, Homi Khusrokhan was MD of Tata Tea. He just took over from Mr. Kidwai. Before settling down in Calcutta, he travelled frequently from Mumbai. In the letter of appreciation that he wrote to me he mentioned that he went to Calcutta on a particular morning. When he was about to leave for Tata Tea's Calcutta office, he saw our literally colorful audit report on his desk. Standing there he started leafing through the pages, then sat down and completed the report at one go! He was late to office!

That was one of the best appreciations we had received for our WDA assignments. Khusrokhan's letter was displayed in the following year's AGMM of the Group to show the importance and effectiveness of our assignment to Group companies.

Information about our WDA assignments for Tata companies reached many quarters. I received requests from some large public sector companies to take up WDA assignments for them. However, we could not accept those offers. We were a small in-house organization.

Apart from WTO related assignments for Tata Group companies, we also did some assignments for apex chambers of commerce of certain government bodies including the Ministry of Commerce. One such project was a 'Tata Memorandum on WTO Compatibility of India's Export Promotion Schemes', prepared in DES under my close supervision, by Jahangir, Sarita and Tanvi. It was hand delivered to Mr. Murasoli Maran, then Minister of Commerce on February 4, 2002. In brief, our study found that most of our export subsidies were non-compatible to WTO norms. The ministry should do something about it. The Minister personally called Dr. Mehta to congratulate and thank for this yeomen work.

We knew if we gave *suo moto* suggestions, usually the establishment would not do anything about it. If our exports grew in a big way in the future, some country some day may take up the issue of the WTO non-compatibility of our export subsidy measures with the WTO. It would be difficult to defend then.

With Jahangir, I did yet another novel study for Tata Motors Ltd (then TELCO) on World Harmonization of Vehicle Regulations and their Convergence with WTO Issues. The study was presented in a seminar organized by Society of Indian Automobile Manufacturers (SIAM), Delhi on August 20, 2002 before the members and guests and senior officials of Surface Transport Ministry, Government of India. Surprisingly, the concerned circles in the country did not know that there were two Working Parties, 1958 and 1998, on harmonization of vehicle regulations and it was important to join one of the working parties.

We prepared large number of notes on topical economic issues. For example, every Friday evening at 4 p.m. we used to mail a one page colorful note, '*The Week That Was*' (with due courtesy to *BBC*).

One Friday, I was in Munnar, Kerala for WTO awareness program. The officer who was coordinating my program, requested me to join him in his office in the evening. When I entered, I saw, to my delight, a dozen PC screens displaying the DES note, '*The Week That Was!*' They told me that the note was a great hit with them.

Sad but true, a bad economy is indeed good for economists. There was such an occasion when an industrial slow down hit us in 1998–99 and continued for a few years. That kept us busy in preparing many company and product specific notes.

In February 2000, Prime Minister Vajpayee established the National Statistical Commission for the first time in the country. Dr. Mehta was one of the members of the Commission, headed by Dr. C.R. Rangarajan, then Governor, Andhra Pradesh. Dr. Mehta deputed me to represent him in the Commission. Representing Dr. Mehta, I actively participated in all 15 working meetings, each for about two full days, of the commission. Dr. Mehta attended a couple of meetings and then, of course the last one, which was the signing by members for sending the report of recommendations to the Prime Minister. I was included in a number of sub-committees – on services, infrastructure and industry, commerce and corporate sector as well as price statistics. It was a wonderful learning as well as networking opportunity for me. I also made my contributions during deliberations.

My areas of interest widened profusely. I had to travel very frequently during that time. Almost twice every week, I was in Delhi for various corporate assignments.

I became a delegate of WTO's well-known Doha Ministerial Meeting during November 9 to 14, 2001. The ministerial meet was a revelation for me to see how laboriously international deals or treaties were made. That exposure helped me to do a better job for on WTO related assignments. I also witnessed the formal entry of the Communist China, which willingly adopted the 'Socialist Market Economy', into the WTO as a member after over 14 years! Literally, there was light, camera, sound all around with hundreds of media persons clicking the shots!

Ironically, that was the time in the historic Doha Ministerial Meet, the whole world was waiting with a batted breath on whether India would say 'NO' to a New Singapore – issues to be included for negotiations in WTO. Saying 'NO' would have nullified WTO's Doha Development Agenda. The meeting was extended by two more days. Doha Sheraton ran out of food. Hardly any delegate left the meeting premises. Saying 'NO' would go against the spirit of the WTO, which was run by 'consensus' only. A 'NO' sayer country could be isolated. Later, everybody was relieved to realize that it perhaps was a negotiating strategy of India. Eventually, a compromise was arrived at to accommodate India's stand and the world breathed a sigh of relief.

While on issues relating to globalization, WTO and the principles of open and free trade, we need to keep in mind that global trade and business are 'adversarially competitive', according to Peter Drucker. There would be both winners and losers. In fact, losers would be more in number than winners. If a country were a loser, the people would suffer. Should a country wait for a backlash? Alternatively, should it introduce a pragmatic people-centric policy? Those were the points for contemplation before formulating a country's growth model as mentioned in the previous chapter.

During that time, many of my papers and articles were published. I also presented my views and opinions in both print and electronic media. I was given the official responsibility to present views on economy and business for the Group. Those were very fulfilling days and I enjoyed sitting on the edge of the chair.

We did a large number of interesting and widely varied assignments during that period with my small team of young and talented economists. Apart from the assignments explained before, we conducted, for example, a study on Kelkar Committee Recommendations on both direct and indirect taxes in December 2002. The team was composed of Jahangir Engineer and Aruna Parimi under my close guidance.

A large number of country specific studies like China, USA, EU, Japan, African and Latin American Countries were also done for the Group companies. Awareness regarding China's increasing business challenge was gathering momentum among the business circles in India. We in DES were closely involved in analyzing developments for the Tata Group.

I was frequently on the move. I attended various meetings, made presentations on specific subjects for the Group or individual companies to ministries, apex chambers of commerce, companies outside Tata Group including certain MNCs like Siemens and a number of embassies.

Besides, many universities and colleges in Mumbai and other cities, Lions and Rotary Clubs in Mumbai, invited me. I was lucky to pack my days, and large part of nights too, with activities. I was lucky to be able to reach so many brains and hearts.

Som and Tapati stood by me; it would not have been possible without their spontaneous support. Tapati went to China in 1997 under ISCCR and CASS international exchange programs for scholars for four weeks to do a research assignment. That was published in 2001 as a book, 'Shanghai and Mumbai: Sustainability of Development in a Globalizing World'. She went to China again in later years and published her second book on China in 2010, 'Yangtze to Ganga: Impact of Economic Reform on Space'.

During that period, Som was doing his MBBS program. By the end of the first year, he suddenly developed a keen interest for playing drums. We bought a full set of drums for him. He and his friends started a band, Zenon, if I remember right. It received good review in the media. He became a proficient drummer. However, after one year, he stopped it and fully concentrated in his studies.

All three of us had been involved in doing something serious. Our life and career moved on. I enjoyed sitting on the edge.

The Phoenix has flown some distance in the sky.

New Horizon

The Western Express Highway is packed with bonnet-to-bonnet traffic even in the middle of the night. I reach home, 18 kms from the airport, after a two-hour crawl on the road. The plane I flew would have covered 1,567 kms in two hours.

It was my privilege to represent the Group Chairman in a full meeting of the Planning Commission held on Monday, February 5, 2001 to present views on growth rates for the economy for the 10th five-year plan (2002–2007). K.C. Pant, Deputy Chairman, was on the chair. The Commission was seeking views of the industry on likely growth rates of the economy and its major sectors. All members and advisers of the commission and many senior industry leaders were present and spoke. I spoke on the prospect of the economy highlighting that it was not the time for setting up a very high 10% average annual rate of growth of GDP in real terms for the 10th plan. With reason and data I explained that 9% or 10%, rate of growth were 'desirable' rates of growth, but not achievable at this stage. At the same time, I appreciated the need for high 9–10% growth rate as the economy could double our per capita GDP in 10 years as China had already done. I mentioned that 9% growth rate of the economy minus 1.8 %, the rate of growth of population, would be equal to 7.2%. The beauty of the number 7.2% was that it doubled in 10 years at compound rate.

That was a wonderful performance by China, no other country could achieve it. It took 32 years for the UK to double its per capita income after second round of industrial revolution from 1830; it took 17 years for the USA from 1870 to 1887 and 15 years for Japan after the World War II. China followed the export-led growth model of Japan to achieve the seemingly impossible task

However, to attain such high rate of growth, the primary sector, which contributed over 27% to GDP in 2001–02, needed to grow at over 4% in a sustainable way. The secondary sector, which contributed about 25% to the GDP in the same year, would have to grow by 8–9%. The tertiary sector, which contributed 48% to the GDP, would have to grow by double digit. The prospect of such high rate of growth had not yet arrived. It was a matter of great satisfaction that the economy had reached the capability of attaining 7.5% to 8% rate of growth for a sustained long period. We must ensure to achieve that feasible rate of growth.

There was a lively discussion after my presentation. I came out with three assignments to be prepared for the commission. They wanted me to send a written version of my talk. One member of Planning Commission, Sompal Shastri, former Cabinet Minister of Agriculture, requested me to write a paper on agriculture. The Deputy Chairman himself requested me for a note on how to make Bihar an investor-friendly state.

I was happy that the important presentation received appreciation.

During that time, I received an all-expenses paid invitation from PMCC, Tokyo and International Simulation and Gaming Association, Kazusa for their 34th annual conference in Japan in August 2003. I did several presentations on the successful completion of the two lead projects, implementation of Cold Rolling Mill (CRM) by Tata Steel in collaboration with Hitachi; and Indica, a passenger car, manufactured by Tata Motors. One of my best treats in Tokyo was an invited dinner at the revolving roof top restaurant. The host was a senior official of the Government of Japan. I shall never forget the warm hospitality that I enjoyed in Japan.

I fondly remembered the story I read in my childhood about four Japanese kids visiting a village in Bengal. They left a great impact on my mind about Japan. My close interactions with my friend Hara in Narendrapur also left many soft ripples about the country, its unique history, culture, its beautiful 'Sakura' – Cherry Blossom. I enjoyed the trip.

Something was prompting me from inside that time was close to make a move. The signal in the mind was louder now. The visit to Japan was a turning point in my life and career. I reached retirement age. There was a strict retirement policy in the group during that period. Under the circumstances, I retired from DES as economic adviser, but continued as a consultant for some time to complete an unfinished study.

My last important work in DES was to direct an empirical study, *'Reforms and Productivity in Indian Manufacturing Sector'* prepared under my close supervision by a small team composed of Raghabendra, Sarita, Dipankar and a statistical consultant Dr. Puspha Trivedi form IIT, Mumbai. The idea of the study originated from a discussion with RG. It was an empirical work, focusing on productivity growth in labor, incremental capital-output ratio (ICOR) as well as total factor productivity (TFP) during pre and post-reform periods. The highlights of the study were published as the centenary publication of the Tata Group in December 2003. Copies were circulated to leaders of the corporate world, government establishments, chambers of commerce and journalists.

Business Standard published major highlights of the study on November 6, 2003, with an editorial by T.N. Ninan Chief Editor. The study covered three sectors – all-India factory sector, top 50 manufacturing companies and six major Tata Group companies. It showed that during the post-reform period there was an improvement in all productivity parameters.[1]

After completing the productivity study, I had certain other ongoing assignments. I did my last WTO Awareness presentation to the top management team of Titan at the company's plant in Hosur, Tamil Nadu, in September 2003. It was the curtain dropping of the WTO initiatives that I had been doing with my team in DES. The drama should have continued for a couple of more acts to reach its logical end. That was not to be as the time bell rang for me.

Over the years, I had been adding value to our corporate assignments of diverse categories, publishing increasing number of papers, taking part in elite seminars and workshops, doing assignments for government bodies, giving interviews to the media and all. I worked hard to elevate

DES as a dynamic economics think tank. I alone could not have done all those, I had a team of young economists to work with me.

I had several bold ideas about our future assignments. If I had five more years, I could have done those assignments with my team. Also, I could have widened further my network among peers, but that's besides the point.

But time had come for the 'Phoenix' to take a turn and glide towards a new horizon.

I had a couple of offers from certain industry quarters. I was thinking about what to do. At the same time, I was sure that I must not stay on as an in-house consultant for long. If you are in the corporate sector, you must be on the driver's seat, in-house consultants are retained for old time's sake. After some time, they are not respected.

Then, one morning I was surprised to get a call from Dr. Manesh Lal Shrikant, Honorary Dean, S.P. Jain Institute of Management & Research (SPJIMR), Mumbai, one of the top management schools in the country. Dr. Shrikant was a visionary educationist and the tallest man in the field of management education in this side of the world. He built SPJIMR as a diversified and reputed management institute as distinguished from a mere business school. He was right in thinking that management education was required not only for business but also for many other sectors of society like government bodies, municipal corporations, police, hospitals and NGOs.

He introduced, inter alia, several 'Beyond Class Room' initiatives in the MBA programs in SPJIMR. That made SPJIMR a unique management school. He was aware that there were many limitations in conventional MBA programs even in the best of business schools in the world. The special initiatives of SPJIMR were to provide a more comprehensive teaching and learning approach.

My joining SPJIMR was coincidental. One young faculty member from SPJIMR, Preeta George, once came to my office in Bombay House for a meeting. Before leaving, she invited me to visit the campus. I received a formal invitation to give a talk to students of SPJIMR on globalization and WTO related issues. Dr. Shrikant attended my talk and handed over a small memento – a silver coin with the name of the institute embossed. He told me that he knew my background and would like me to join his institute after I retired from the Tata Group. I thought that was a just polite and courteous conversation.

Then – after a few years – he called me! I met him the following morning for more than an hour. To cut a long story short, he insisted that I must immediately join the institute as a Professor.

Teaching in a business school was never in my mind. Now I thought why not. I retired from Tata Group after working almost for three decades. I left Bombay House on May 24, 2004. I remembered my first day – February 17, 1975 – in DES, my desk next to peons! I had a heartwarming one to one meeting with Chairman Ratan Tata before my leaving the House. I said goodbye to my team. I said goodbye to Bombay House.

The next day I joined SPJIMR as a Professor. I moved over from a corporate economist to a teacher in a business school and my new learning began. Coming from the corporate sector to an educational institution required some conscious efforts to adjust. I had prepared my mind about it, so there was no problem for adjustment.

Giving a talk on a topic is one thing. However, to teach a full course to MBA students was entirely different. Dr. Shrikant helped me in my learning. I attended sessions conducted by him and some other faculty members, both senior and young. Then I structured my own pedagogue. I taught International Business to all four MBA programs in SPJIMR. I also introduced an elective course on global competitiveness for PGDM participants. Besides, I taught Economics and Business Environment including the '*Economic Times*' (ET) classes, which was Dr. Shrikant's idea. Dr. Pallavi Mody was with me for the ET classes. It was a wonderful experience to work together with experienced teachers. I had no ego problem in learning from any one, senior or young.

On Dr. Shrikant's request, I prepared a framework for teaching and learning a new – Integrated Course – on Ethics and Business. A stand-alone course on Ethics and Business could simply be smiled off as an oxymoron – even if it was delivered by Mark Antony. I prepared a framework based largely on the four-sphere architecture of Prof. J.L. Bodaracco Jr., of Harvard Business School[2] to integrate the teaching and learning of Ethics and Business across all other courses in PGDM. It became a unique course, taught by a number of faculty members.

Alongside teaching and being closely involved in SPJIMR's 'Beyond Classroom Initiatives', I got closely involved in conducting a corporate government research, organizing seminars, courses and round tables on the subject. As an accredited institution of National Foundation of Corporate Governance (NFCG), we had to take up corporate governance initiatives in SPJIMR. Dr. Shrikant left it to me.

I assembled a small team – Prof. Debasis Mallik, Dolly Dhamodiwala, senior researcher, and research associates Manjula Hari Krishan Krishnan, Kirti Rao, Sonali and Pallavi Das – each working during different phases. We conducted a number of empirical research studies on corporate governance, organized seminars, round tables and courses with sponsorship of NFCG. All four of our research reports, three round tables and courses organized by us in SPJIMR could be accessed from the NFCG website.[3] Experts in the field commended our corporate governance initiatives.

Many eminent critics raised points about business school related issues and particular curriculum. Since the 1950s, the development of pedagogue in top business schools in the USA like Harvard Business School (HBS) was case-based teaching and learning. Cases were written largely on manufacturing companies. Those were the glorious days of the American manufacturing sector.

Before raising the issue for discussion, I wrote a case, co-authored with three of my PGDM 2012 batch students. The case was published[4]; it also won a contest. That was to establish my credibility on the subject as teacher in a management school. One point of concern in India was the overemphasis on teaching based on cases, which were very lengthy with irrelevant content and written decades ago. Naturally, they did not connect with the typical Indian business context.

Dr. Shrikant was a superb case teacher. I named specific cases, written decades ago, which were taught for years and years and years. I explained how those contents were irrelevant. He listened to me patiently and left with a smile saying, you teach your international business courses the way you would like to do.

As mentioned, several eminent experts voiced concerns regarding the limitations of management education. To mention just three: Prof. Henry Mintzberg of McGill University Montreal, Canada (since 2009), Prof. Srikant M. Datar of HBS (2010) and very recently Rana Faroohar (2016). Rana Faroohar explained in her book at length about reforming the B-school curriculum. She observed with examples that a wave of 'financialization' had taken over the core of the global business, generating new and complex dynamics.[5]

During recent years, businesses have massively changed. More than half of the US manufacturing has moved out to China as discussed in an earlier chapter. There has been huge growth of the heterogeneous services sector, including information technology services. Over 80% of the US GDP comes from the services sector.

Over and above, the future business is now poised for the growth of digital technology, three-D production, artificial intelligence, robotics and nano technology. There are changes and disruptions every moment. These dynamics will be faster and more volatile in the future. These are going to dominate the business arena. The changing time, the typical nature and characteristics of Indian business demands curriculum and pedagogic innovations in our management education.

Encouragingly, there are enough evidence of the availability of managerial talent and expertise in the country. For example, the efficient organization of the *Kumbh Mela* with millions of people visiting, staying for a few days and bathing, did not require any foreign-trained management experts. On a humble scale, the smooth and hassle free operation of Dabbawalas in Mumbai, supplying food to office goers every day did not require foreign-trained management experts. Take also the running of giant kitchens in certain parts of India, shown by National Geographic channels, efficiently supplying food to thousands of people every day.

Besides, there are many illustrious industrialists and managers in the country, who never went to any business school or learnt management expertise. Based on my decades' long working experience in the Tata Group, it is my considered view that we can develop the desired curriculum and pedagogue for management education for India from the available expertise and strength of our own.

It is time for my second retirement – this time from SPJIMR after working as Professor for over 13 years. Has time come for me to take a pause, stretch my legs up, and watch the Sunset? Well, certainly not. I have been comfortable sitting on the edge of the chair. For me work is life. The model of so-called work-life balance is not for me. To my mind, you cannot compartmentalize the two.

I got involved in doing some consultancy works on honorary basis and writing. While doing all this, I received, surprisingly, an invitation from my friend Dr. Harshvardhan Halve, director, Jaipuria Institute of Management, Indore (JIM-I). JIM-I is the youngest of the three older business schools located in Lucknow, Jaipur and Noida. He is passionate about making JIM-I a top business school in Central India. He discussed with me the possibility of creating and conducting some innovative and experiential teaching/ learning pedagogue for his students.

On his request, I joined JIM, Indore as adjunct faculty. I applied my mind, architecture – and successfully conducted – two courses (one credit each) through non-classroom, i.e. workshop modes. The courses are Ethics & Governance, and Business & Sustainable Development. I also conducted a workshop for faculty members on review of management education in Indian business schools.

Teaching these courses through conventional classroom mode is not effective at all. I have already mentioned this. The new experiential mode turned out to be relevant and useful. After the workshop, students write a diary, narrating how their mind moved across the course track from the beginning to the end. Take a random selection of these diaries, you would find that the essence of the learning has reached young students.

I go to the beautiful campus of JIM-I as and when required. I find that Central Indian students are aspiring; both teachers and staff members are fully committed and the management takes care. JIM-I has received several accreditations and ratings. I believe it has a great future. I feel good to be involved here.

It was my overwhelming satisfaction to interact with students. As faculty in charge of certain committees in SPJIMR, it was my pleasure to personally know and interact with many of them. Supervising their reports, discussing their questions, deliberating on current issues, off class room discussions, guiding them for inter-business school competitions, supporting them organize the institutes' cultural-cum academic fests, building bridges with the Tata Group gave me a wonderful opportunity and exposure to know, and reach out to, these young students. I was happy to be able to establish a 'connect' with the young brain and mind. I know they also value this relationship.

It was satisfying to interact with colleagues during hearty and freewheeling '*Adda*' over tea and *samosa,* discussing 'Cabbages and Kings'. I was faculty in-charge of the institute's library; it enhanced my reading. The touch, feel and smell of new books always gave me joy.

It is important, in this context, to reiterate here about my relationship with my former teenaged students of Narendrapur school. They needed to be treated with sufficient degree of love, affection, care as well as with firmness when required. Over the years, this warm relationship has become deep and sustaining. When I started teaching on the side since 1962, I was a first year student in Economics Honors class. Thus, our age difference was not much. By now, they have retired; some have become grandfathers! They are my extended family. They have made my life joyous and rewarding.

I conclude this chapter sharing my experience relating my exposure to a Chinese business school. I received an invitation from Business School of Lioning University, Shenyang, China to give a talk in the inaugural session of their MBA Day in November 2012. I also had discussion meetings with the senior officers of China Academy of Social Science (CASS) in Beijing.

Since college days, I had been closely studying and following developments in China for a long time. In my working life, I prepared many studies on China. In my international business classes, Chinese experiences were important to study. The trip therefore was very fulfilling. I shall always remember the warm hospitality that I received in Shenyang and Beijing.

Epilogue

'The best view comes after the hardest climb.'

Life moves on. The next generation and their children arrived and started moving at a faster pace. They would reach greater heights. The third generation would live and work in a high-tech digital world, strikingly different from ours. They would be the real Jonathan Livingston Seagulls, for whom there would not be any 'Limits'.

In my life, I have encountered many giants among men and women, indeed with large and warm hearts. I have been happy to come across people who are wise and compassionate to others. They make this world a beautiful place.

It was exultant for me to engage with many so called ordinary people having gorgeous minds and hearts. They are simple, plain speaking, functionally wise and honest. They are gems among us.

I am distressed to see pompous, vain, and harmful people occupying high places. History has it that they have divided and broken countries, started war among people and nations, killing and uprooting millions. I am disturbed to see many ambitious, rich and wealthy, albeit greedy people. They do not know when and where to stop. They have not learned the virtue of *Aprigarh*. They made themselves miserable. They even do not know that.

"All the world is a stage, And all the men and women merely players. They have exits and their entrances," said William Shakespeare. I have encountered many of them in my life. They made my journey exciting, lively and interesting.

I must mention here what a respected teacher told me once. He said howsoever materially successful you are in life, unless you receive love and respect from your own children, your success is just apparent. As parents, we are overwhelmingly happy to receive love and respect of our son.

As a teacher, I sincerely tried to mentor the 'live young elements' (my words) – the students! It was challenging and fulfilling. I feel happy that I have been able to reach the heart and brain of my students. My students from SPJIMR and JIM-I are young; they are amidst climbing up steps on the ladder of their lives and careers.

Many of my students from Narendrapur have lived a wholesome life. Some are established names in their respective professions. They are my extended family. What more reward could I expect from life!

As persons, we in the family – Tapati, Som and I – always did our best to reach out to our friends, relatives as well as the community to try to be with them in their times of tears and joy. Sometimes someone could be hit hard in life. Usually it happens, randomly, all of a sudden. That is the time they need a helping hand. We try to be around.

In a story, a mother with a dead child in her arms comes to Gautama Buddha and begs him to bring the child back to life. Buddha asks her to go to the city to get a fistful of mustard from a family that had not seen suffering of any kind. Once she brings it, Buddha says, he will give life back to the child. The mother is relieved initially as she thinks it will be an easy task. She goes for the entire day from house to house, but finds no such family in the city that has not suffered with sickness, accident or death.

Times of tears are the time when you need a genuine, warm and friendly hand to hold. We have tried our humble best to be around in such cases. We have also received help when we suffered. Life moves on smoothly by holding each others' hands.

There could be mass death and destruction in war, natural calamity or manmade disasters – like the one we suffered during Partition.

In this journey across time and space, many people have been with and around me. Some said goodbye and got down when their respective destinations arrived. Some moved in with good wishes and camaraderie. Though I have been with them in different stretches of this long journey, internally I remained essentially alone.

In fact, I have been travelling this world like a roving 'Outsider'.

Notes

Preface

1. The Concise Oxford Dictionary, Oxford University Press.
2. SPARK Notes, www.sparknotes.com/lit/ulysses/context.html

Chapter 2

1. Bikrampurer Itihas (in Bengali), CHAPTER 5various chapters, edited by Kamal Choudhary, Dey's Publications, Calcutta 2004
2. Ibid
3. Antarjwali Jatra, published in 'Upanyas Samagra' (Collected Novels in Bengali), Kamal Kumar Mazumdar, Anand Publishers, 2014

Chapter 3

1. BBC – India's Partition: The Forgotten Story 2017, a documentary by Gurinder Chadha

Chapter 5

1. A popular Hindi proverb, meaning: Travelers, pack your bags, you have a long way to go.
2. Thirty-two *Kathas* make one Acre, or one *Katha* is equal to 67 sq meters.
3. Debadatta Chaudhury, Space, Identity, Territory: Marichjhapi Massacre, 1979, The International Journal of Human Rights, Vol. 15, 2011, Issue 5.

Chapter 6

1. National Aeronautics & Space Administration, NASA Science Brief, John Knox, April 1997

Chapter 8

1. Based on Chinese Embassy in India (in.chineseembassy.org)
2. A Life in Diplomacy, Maharajakrishna Rasgotra, China's Warnings of War, Chapter 12, Penguin Books India, 2016, Chapter 12, p 81.

Chapter 9

1. Dark Nature: A Natural History of Evil, Lyall Watson, Harper Collins, NY, 1995

Chapter 11

1. There are a few websites for the ashram, school, college, Lokashiksha Parishad of Ramakrishna Mission Ashram, Narendrapur. Interested reader may visit them to get a detailed picture.
2. Ideology of Ramakrishna Math and Mission, (www.belurmath. org/ideology.htm)

Chapter 13

1. Calcutta Diary, Ashok Mitra, published by Pranajoy Guha Thakurta,

Chapter 14

1. The Two Year Mountain by Phil Deutschle, Bradt, 1986
2. op. cit. SPARK

Chapter 15

1. Statistical Outline of India, Department of Economics and statistics, Tata Services Ltd, 2014–15, Tables 2, 3 and 4

Chapter 17

1. *What Should I Do with My life?* Po Bronson, Vintage Book, 2002

Chapter 18

1. *Many Lives, Many Masters*, Dr. Brian Weiss, first published in 1988
2. *Through Time Into Healing* (*How Past Life Regression Therapy can Heal Mind and Soul*), Dr. Brian Weiss, 1992... and six other books
3. www.nobelprize.org/nobel_prize/literature/1964/pres.htm
4. *The Stranger*, Albert Camus, 1942
5. *Waiting for Godot*, a play by Samuel Beckett, Grover Press

Chapter 19

1. Population Explosion in West Bengal, A Survey done by South Asia Research Society, Calcutta, quoting data from Economic Review 1971–72, Government of West Bengal The Economist, September 12, 2015
2. *The Economist*, May 28, 2016, Special Report on Migration, p 4.
3. The World Fact Book, CIA
4. Millennium Development Goals, Bangladesh Progress Report, Planning Commission, 2015

Chapter 20

1. The author calculated data on election results from various reports from the Election Commission of India.
2. *Indira: The Life of Indira Gandhi*, Katherine Frank, Houghton Mifflin Harcourt, 2002
3. *The Maoist Insurgency in Nepal...*, Lawti, Mahendra, et al, Routlege, p 206, 2009
4. Data on Lok Sabha Election results of 2014 from Election Commission of India. Also, consulted West Bengal Lok Sabha History (www.elections.in/west-bengal/parliamentary-constituencies)

Chapter 22

1. The Official Website of Purulia District (www.purulia.nic.in)
2. Ibid, The Official Website of Purulia District

Chapter 23

1. West Bengal Development Report, Planning Commission, Government of India, published by Academic Foundation, p 63
2. Department of Industrial Promotion and Policy (DIPP), Government of India (web site: dipp.nic.in)
3. Ibid, DIPP (State – wise Statistics on Investment Proposals in 2015, 2016, February 2017)
4. Ananda Bazar Patrika March 11, 2019
5. Made in the USA, The Rise and Retreat of American Manufacturing, Vaclav Smil, MIT Press, 2013

Chapter 26

1. *150-Yr-old Heritage in Concrete Jungle*, Ruhi Bhasin, The Indian Express, Mumbai, February 6 2017, p 5

Chapter 28

1. *The Creation of Wealth*, R.M. Lala, 2004 edition, Viking, Penguin India, p.88

Chapter 29

1. The Economic Survey, Ministry of Finance, Government of India, 1991–92, Payments Crisis, pp 10–11.
2. The Economic Survey, Ministry of Finance, Government of India 1992–93, p117
3. *Half-Lion: How P V Narasimha Rao Transformed India*, Vinay Sitapati, Viking, 2016, Chapter 7.
4. 1091: How Narasimha Rao Made History, Sanjaya Baru, 2016
5. CIA, *The World Fact Book*, February 2018

Chapter 31

1. Reforms and Productivity Trends in Manufacturing Sector, A Study by Department of Economics and statistics, Tata services Ltd, Mumbai, Project Director, Jiban K Mukhopadhyay, December 2003.
2. Prof. J.L. Bodaracco, Business Ethics: Role and Responsibilities, HBSP, 1995
3. www.nfcg.in
4. *A Case on RLEK: Survival with the Bottom Line*, by Jiban K Mukhopadhyay with Mayank Garg, Saumya Oli and Arun Kumar (PGDM batch 2012 SPJIMR), published by Ivey(9B12M029), 2012, won a contest organized by ISB-Ivey.
5. *Makers and Takers: How Wall Street Destroyed Main Street*, Rana Faroohar, Crown Business, New York, 2016

✳✳✳

Lightning Source UK Ltd.
Milton Keynes UK
UKHW010934270722
406450UK00001B/31

9 781645 871668